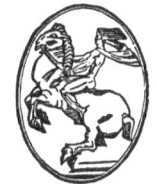

VIROLOGY MONOGRAPHS

DIE VIRUSFORSCHUNG IN EINZELDARSTELLUNGEN

CONTINUATION OF / FORTFÜHRUNG VON
HANDBOOK OF VIRUS RESEARCH
HANDBUCH DER VIRUSFORSCHUNG
FOUNDED BY / BEGRÜNDET VON
R. DOERR

EDITED BY / HERAUSGEGEBEN VON

S. GARD · C. HALLAUER

15

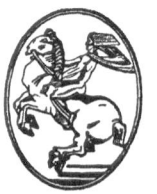

1976

SPRINGER-VERLAG

WIEN   NEW YORK

THE PARVOVIRUSES

BY

G. SIEGL

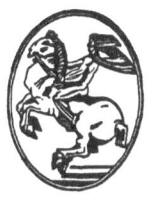

1976

SPRINGER-VERLAG

WIEN   NEW YORK

ISBN-13: 978-3-7091-8432-5   e-ISBN-13: 978-3-7091-8430-1
DOI: 10.1007/978-3-7091-8430-1

The Parvoviruses

By

Günter Siegl

Institute of Hygiene and Medical Microbiology,
University of Bern, Bern, Switzerland

With 1 Figure

Table of Contents

I. Introduction

Parvoviruses belong to the large group of viral agents of which virologists have become aware by chance in many biological materials due to the availability of more sensitive isolation techniques and the extensive use of the electron microscope. In general, many of these viruses lacked the stimulating background of an infectious disease and, therefore, have fallen into oblivion already soon after discovery. In case of parvoviruses, however, interest has been maintained because of the circumstances under which most of them were isolated.

A great number of parvoviruses has been recovered from tissues of tumor-bearing animals, from cell-free filtrates of tumors, or from stable cell lines of tumor origin. These observations necessarily suggested the newly isolated viral agents of playing an important, yet unknown role in the induction and development of cancer. On the other hand, further parvoviruses were found constantly associated with adenoviruses. It was the experimental analysis of the multiplication behaviour which then revealed that the association between parvoviruses and tumors or parvoviruses and adenoviruses originates from the basis of a certain genetic defectiveness. For some members of the group this may be overcome by cellular helper effects in rapidly growing tissues, for several others, however, by biochemical events in the simultaneously occurring replication of an adenovirus only.

Additional points of view in favour of parvovirus research have arisen from experimental animal studies. Although the majority of the viruses persist as latent infections in their natural hosts, inoculation of certain strains into newborn hamsters resulted in a broad variety of syndromes including osteolysis, ataxia, and mongoloid-like features. Moreover, congenital malformations developed following infection during pregnancy. Since similar syndromes are well known to occur also under natural conditions in animals and man, parvoviruses have been supposed to play the role of etiologic agents. At present, however, only feline cerebellar ataxia could be shown to result from infection with the specific parvovirus of felines which, besides that, had been identified previously as the cause of feline panleukopenia and mink enteritis.

A final reason why parvoviruses attracted the interest of virologists may be found in the fact that the group comprises the smallest animal DNA viruses so far known. The viral particles consist of nothing but an isometric protein capsid and a short molecule of single-stranded DNA sufficient to code for 3 to 5 proteins only. Such a small number of viral genes suggests parvoviruses to present an ideal experimental system for the study of biochemical processes occurring in course of the replication of DNA viruses. Moreover, parvoviruses have put forward the question how a single-stranded DNA is replicated in an eukaryotic cell.

In the following chapters emphasis is placed on the characteristics of those members of the genus parvovirus (cf. Table 1) which are able to multiply in vertebrate cells without assistance of a potent helper virus. For precise information on the fully defective adeno-associated viruses as well as on densonucleosis virus, the so far only parvovirus isolated from an insect, the reader is referred to the excellent reviews of HOGGAN (1970, 1971) and KURSTAK (1972), respectively.

II. Nomenclature and Classification

Both in size and morphology the viruses dealt with in the present report resemble the smallest RNA viruses, the picornaviruses. When reviewing the characteristics of the newly isolated agents, MAYOR and MELNICK (1966) therefore felt that this property and the DNA nature of the nucleic acid would justify their denotation as *picodna*viruses in analogy to the term picorna (pico = very small, RNA). At the time when the nucleic acid of the helper-independent small DNA viruses was found to be a single-stranded, whereas the DNA of the adenoassociated viruses appeared to be a double-stranded molecule, the International

Table 1. *Classification of Parvoviruses*

Family *Parvoviridae*

Genus *Parvovirus*

Type species: Parvovirus r-1 (rat virus)

Member viruses:
    Rat virus (RV)
    H-1 virus
    Minute virus of mice (MVM)
    Porcine parvovirus (PPV)
    Bovine parvovirus (BPV)
    Feline parvovirus (FPV)
    TVX
    Lu III
    RTV

Possible members:
    Canine parvovirus (MVC)
    Goose hepatitis virus
    Hepatitis A virus of man
    Gastroenteritis virus of man

Genus *Adeno-Associated Virus*

Type species: AAV type 1

Member viruses:
    AAV type 1
    AAV type 2
    AAV type 3
    AAV type 4
    Bovine AAV (X 7)
    Avian AAV (AAAV)

Possible member:
    Canine AAV

Genus *Densovirus*

Type species: Densonucleosis virus *(galleria)*

Member virus:
    Densonucleosis virus

Possible member:
    Junonia virus

Committee on the Nomenclature of Viruses (ICNV), however, accepted the name parvoviruses (from parvus = small) to cover the whole group.

Membership in the parvovirus group is based on physicochemical characteristics. The viruses are isometric, non enveloped particles with a diameter of 18 to 26 nm. Their capsid, probably constructed of 32 capsomeres, shows icosahedral symmetry and encloses a single-stranded, linear DNA having a molecular weight of between 1.2 to 2.0×10^6 daltons. Moreover, the viruses band at densities between 1.38 to 1.47 g/ml in CsCl, sediment with about 110 Svedberg units, resist the action of ether, and are stable to heating at 56° C.

In the majority of the parvoviruses isolated so far, the infective particle contains only one type of single-stranded DNA. In others, however, complementary single-strands are separately encapsidated which, upon extraction, anneal spontaneously *in vitro* to form a double-stranded molecule. These characteristics and the fact that some of the members of the parvovirus group multiply only in the presence of an adenovirus helper currently has been used to divide the family *Parvoviridae* into three genera (Table 1):

(i) The genus **Parvovirus** comprises all viruses which encapsidate only one type of single-stranded DNA* and multiply without the help of an adenovirus. At present, 9 viruses representing 9 different serotypes have been definitely included by the ICNV. Possible additional members are the minute virus of canines (MVC), goose hepatitis virus, hepatitis A virus of man, and the virus causing acute nonbacterial gastroenteritis of man.

(ii) Replication of members of the genus **Adeno-Associated Virus** (AAV) depends upon helper viruses. Moreover, the single strands of the DNA incorporated by individual particles are complementary. Six serotypes have been admitted to the genus and the canine adeno-associated virus is regarded as a potential member.

(iii) At present, the genus **Densovirus** is restricted to the densonucleosis virus (DNV), a parvovirus isolated from *Galleria mellonella, L.* and to Junonia virus as a possible member. DNV replicates without a helper virus; yet, the single strands of the DNA are complementary and, upon extraction, form a double-stranded DNA *in vitro*.

III. Properties of Parvoviruses

Viruses classified within the genus Parvovirus of the family *Parvoviridae* share identical physicochemical characteristics with members of the genus Adeno-Associated Virus and the genus Densovirus (cf. Nomenclature and Classification, and Table 7). In contrast to viruses enclosed in the latter two genera, however, they all agglutinate red blood cells of at least one species (cf. Table 8). Moreover, these viruses are capable of multiplying in susceptible cells without being supported by the simultaneous replication of a helper virus. The obviously limited genetic information of their nucleic acid nevertheless has to be complemented by specific functions displayed only shortly during the lifecycle of an infected cell.

---

* See addendum.

Both *in vitro* and *in vivo* multiplication of parvoviruses, therefore, is restricted to tissues supplying a large amount of cells undergoing mitosis and, furthermore, all clinico-pathologic syndromes observed so far in consequence to infections with these viruses could be traced back to the dependence of virus multiplication on cellular physiology.

In spite of this obvious homogeneity, the characteristics in common to the individual members of the genus parvovirus shall not be presented in comprehensive chapters. Such an attempt would result either in an undue loss of information or in an extended, unintelligible summation of data. To provide both clarity and information, the various viruses have been grouped as far as possible with reference to their source of isolation (*i. e.* mainly their natural host). This should enable the reader to inform quickly on a certain agent without working through the whole article.

A. Hamster-Osteolytic Viruses and Related Isolates

1. History

The name "hamster-osteolytic viruses" specifies several viral isolates which for many years have been distinguished from other parvoviruses by their exceptional pathogenicity for newborn hamsters. Their discovery by KILHAM and OLIVIER (1959) and TOOLAN (1960) also is equivalent to the beginning of our knowledge on the whole parvovirus group. One of the hamster-osteolytic agents — Kilham rat virus (RV) — has been chosen as the type species of the genus *Parvovirus*.

RV owes its discovery to the search for an anticipated papovavirus of rats. When during the course of these investigations KILHAM and OLIVIER (1959) inoculated tumor tissue homogenates from three rats of the Fisher and Osborne-Mendel strain bearing either spontaneous liver sarcomas associated with encysted cat tapeworm larvae *(Cysticercus fasciolaris)* or a transplantable rat leukemia (DUNNING and CURTIS, 1957) into rat embryonic cell cultures, they were able to isolate a virus with certain resemblance to the papovaviruses: It multiplied and induced cytopathogenic alterations in cultures of embryonic rat cells, agglutinated both guinea pig and rat erythrocytes, and resisted ether treatment as well as heating to 80° C for 2 hours. In contrast to the papovaviruses, however, RV apparently lacked oncogenicitiy and — at that early stage of investigation — proved to be apathogenic for newborn or weanling rats, suckling mice and hamsters, as well as for adult guinea pigs and rabbits.

In contrast to the then apparently apathogenic behaviour of RV, the H-viruses attracted special attention by the distinctive malformations they induced in newborn hamsters. The deformities became evident for the first time when TOOLAN (1960a) injected fractions of various transplantable human tumors (HEp-1, HEp-3, HEp-4, HEp-5, HS-1, HEmb Rh-1, HAd-1, A-42) into neonates and consisted in dwarfism, flat face, microcephalic domed head, protruding eyes and tongue, fragility of bones and malformation or complete absence of teeth. Soon afterwards (TOOLAN *et al.*, 1960) the possibility to reproduce these abnormalities even after inoculation of cell-free filtrates of both the original transplantable tumors and tissues obtained from affected hamsters already suggested the causative agent to be a virus. This hypothesis could be ascertained when electron microscopic examination of samples originating from the transplantable human tumor HEp-1 revealed the presence of small virus particles measuring only 15—30 nm in diameter. Referring to its source, the isolated agent was named H-1.

Before the successful isolation of H-1 virus from HEp-1 cells, this human tumor has been serially transplanted in cortisone-treated as well as X-irradiated rats. A similar method of continuous passage in rats was used to maintain the human tumor HEp-3 from which DALLDORF (1960) after transferring it to hamsters recovered a virus with H-1 characteristics, later on referred to as H-3 (sometimes also OLV). When, therefore, KILHAM (1961 a, b) recorded the presence of specific neutralizing antibodies to RV in sera of a large number of laboratory rats and—in contrast to earlier findings (KILHAM and OLIVIER, 1959)—observed the development of dwarfism and related deformities after injection of the agent into newborn hamsters, there arose the question whether RV, H-1, and H-3 virus might be identical. Subsequent cross neutralization tests then revealed a close serologic relationship existing between RV and H-3, and hence, could not exclude the possibility that H-3 was picked up from rats during continuous transplantation of the HEp-3 tumor in animals of this species. H-1 virus, on the other hand, proved to be serologically unrelated to both RV and H-3 virus.

The recovery of H-1 and H-3 virus after inoculation of human tumors into newborn hamsters as well as the spectrum of malformations observed in the animals of course also suggested the question for the significance of these agents in human disease. Further isolation attempts were undertaken and—according to the original experimental results—the use of human neoplastic and embryonic tissues as a potent source for virus isolations looked very promising. Presence or absence of virus was again demonstrated by inoculating fractions of the suspicious tissues into hamster neonates. During these studies H-1 virus then could be recovered from various tissues of cancer patients (TOOLAN 1961 a, b) as well as from two out of eight human embryos (TOOLAN et al., 1962). Occurrence of another virus, HT, apparently serologically related to but not completely identical with H-1, was also demonstrated in human embryos and, in addition, was found present in placentas (TOOLAN, 1964). At the same time TOOLAN (1964) also reported the isolation of HB-virus from a cystadenocarcinoma of the ovary of a twelve-year old girl, from one human embryo, and from two placentas. The latter agent proved to be serologically unrelated both to H-1 and RV.

So far, agents serologically related to or even identical with RV could only be isolated from rat tissues. The circumstances of most of these isolations share several additional characteristic features in common, since the respective viruses usually were recovered from rats either bearing tumors or treated with X-rays and/or chemical substances. In contrast to the methods used by TOOLAN (1960 a, b) and TOOLAN et al. (1961), the RV-like agents were detected in the harvests of primary and secondary rat-embryonic cell cultures inoculated with suspicious tissue homogenates. Using this technique, PAYNE et al. (1963) became aware of X-14 virus in mammary tissues of an X-irradiated and methyl-cholanthrene-treated Sprague-Dawley rat and LUM and SCHREINER (1963) recovered the LS-agent from a Wistar rat chloroleukemic tumor. At that very time LS-virus was unique among the other isolates in being apparently apathogenic for hamster neonates. Soon afterwards, however, KILHAM and MOLONEY (1964) reported the isolation of one RV-strain with similar characteristics from tissues of rats inoculated with Moloney leukemia virus. It is known that these two virus strains may cause cerebellar hypoplasia and ataxia when injected intracerebrally into newborn hamsters (LUM, 1970). In two other instances, presence of RV could be demonstrated in rats with leukemia induced by application of high doses of dimethylbenzanthrene (SPENCER, 1967) and injection of rat mammary tumor extracts (BERGS, 1967), respectively. This close association between the incidence of neoplasms and the occurrence of demonstrable RV-infection also became evident when ZHDANOV and MEREKALOVA (1962) were able to isolate the so-called Krisini-virus from connective tissue of rats treated with carcinogens. According to FERM and KILHAM (1964), this agent resembles RV and H-3 virus both serologically and in its pathogenicity for hamsters.

This picture of rat virus infection suggested by the above cited observations was put in the proper perspective when numerous experimental *in vivo* and *in vitro* studies proved a close relationship between successful virus multiplication and an elevated mitotic activity of susceptible cells. Moreover, screening for specific antibodies in sera collected from both wild and laboratory rats yielded positive results in about 80 per cent of the tested samples and thus reflected an extremely high prevalence of RV infections in rat colonies (MOORE and NICASTRI, 1965; KILHAM, 1966; NATHANSON and COLE, 1968). According to ROBEY *et al.* (1968) who tested rats of different laboratory strains for both presence of specific antibody to RV and the possibility to isolate the virus from various tissues of animals in susceptible cell cultures, presence of demonstrable antibody is also equivalent to the status of a persistent, latent RV-infection. It was concluded from all these observations that the process of tumor induction in rats, in close resemblance to the highly susceptible embryonic tissues, provides an elevated number of actively dividing cells and, thus, the possibility to convert a latent RV-infection into a frank one. In this respect, a further important factor—*i.e.* an immunological one—became evident when EL DADAH and coworkers (1967) treated apparently healthy rats of a colony in which RV-infection was prevalent with the immuno-suppressive drug cyclophosphamide. About two per cent of the animals showed paralysis of the hind limbs within two to three weeks after injection. A virus serologically related to RV was recovered from brain and spinal cord of these animals and intracerebral inoculation of the agent in suckling rats regularly resulted in acute fatal paralysis associated with hemorrhages and necroses in the brain and spinal cord. Consistent with the specific syndrome this RV-strain was referred to as the "hemorrhagic encephalopathy of rats (HER-) agent".

More recently, parvoviruses related to the hamster-osteolytic agents have been identified as contaminants in various tissue culture studies. MELNICK *et al.* (1971) recovered a parvovirus with the antigenic characteristics of H-3 virus from a cloned line of Detroit-6 cells (neoplastic human bone marrow) after inoculation of human plasma known to contain hepatitis A virus and BERQUIST *et al.* (1972) demonstrated the presence of a very similar virus in human embryonic lung (HEL) cell cultures infected with stool specimens of children suffering from type A hepatitis. In both cases, however, evidence could be obtained that the isolated viruses were not related to the etiologic agent of human hepatitis.

HALLAUER and coworkers (1971), on the other hand, reported the isolation of a parvovirus (RTV) from a permanent line of embryonic rat cells (AT) originally established by P. Tournier. With reference to its source the agent was termed RT-virus. It proved to be pathogenic for newborn hamsters and showed a host cell range limited to cells of rat and hamster origin. No serologic relationship to any of the other known parvoviruses could be established so far.

2. Morphology

a) Size

First evidence for the size of the hamster-osteolytic viruses was obtained from ultrahistological studies centred on the multiplication of H-1 virus in tissues of infected hamsters. Both in liver Kupffer cells and in interstitial kidney cells of 3 to 11 day old animals inoculated within 24 hours after birth, CHANDRA and TOOLAN (1961) observed large groups of particles characterized by a heavy staining 15 nm sized core and regularly separated from each other by an approximately 7.5 nm wide electron-lucent space. The particles readily could be distinguished from ribosomes. Referring to the electron-lucent zone as an integral, but—by means of the fixation and staining techniques used—only insufficiently characterized part of the morphological entity, the authors finally suggested the maximum overall diameter of H-1 to be 30 nm. Further electron microscopic investigations on cells infected either *in vivo* or *in vitro* by H-1, RV, as well as X-14 virus confirmed the observation that, in ultrathin sections, the clearly demonstrable core of the hamster-osteolytic viruses measures 13 to 18 nm in diameter (BERNHARD et al., 1963; DALTON et al., 1963; MAYOR and JORDAN, 1966; RUFFALO et al., 1966; AL-LAMI et al., 1969). As DALTON et al. (1963) pointed out, this value represents only half the figure of 35 nm determined during ultrahistological examinations of the core of polyoma- and K-virus and, yet, refuted the membership of the hamster-osteolytic viruses within the papova-virus group then still assumed by KILHAM (1961a, b). Electron microscopy of purified, unconcentrated virus suspensions stained by the negative contrast method provides an easier means of estimating the overall size of particles than did ultrasectioning of infected cells. The reliability of values obtained in this way, however, depends on the extent to which preparation methods and working conditions of the electron microscope influence flattening or preservation of the agent's shape. The diameters recorded for the hamster-osteolytic viruses in various laboratories—20 to 29 nm (TOOLAN et al., 1964), 23 ± 2 nm (GREEN and KARASAKI, 1965), and 30 ± 1.5 nm (McGEOGH et al., 1970) for H-1; 20 nm (BREESE et al., 1964), 18 ± 1.5 nm (VASQUEZ and BRAILOVSKY, 1965), 18 nm (MAY et al., 1967), 22 nm (WHITMAN and HETRICK, 1967), and 28 ± 1 nm (McGEOCH et al., 1970) for RV; 18—24 nm (PAYNE et al., 1964), 20 nm (JAMISON and MAYOR, 1965), and 22 nm (MAYOR and JORDAN, 1966) for X-14, as well as 19—21 nm for RT-virus (SIEGL et al., unpublished)—therefore reflect nothing but the fact that these agents range in size between 18 to 30 nm. Much more meaningful in respect to the possibility that different strains of the hamster-osteolytic viruses may vary in size are the results of KARASAKI (1966) who estimated the diameters of RV, H-1, H-3, HT, and HB virus under constant and controlled experimental conditions. The additional use of specific antisera to obtain large agglomerations of virus particles from diluted suspensions thereby also revealed that, in parallel to the serologic relationship, the viruses may be grouped according to their size. Both H-1 and HT virus were 21.5 ± 2 nm in diameter, whereas H-3 and RV only measured 19 ± 2 nm. The serologically unrelated HB-virus could be grouped with RV and H-3.

b) Structure

In accordance with their proved resistance to the action of lipid solvents, the hamster-osteolytic viruses are devoid of an envelope. Negative staining gave rise to the appearance of both "empty" and "full" particles, the central dark space of the empty ones with a diameter of 12 to 15 nm (TOOLAN et al., 1964; VASQUEZ and BRAILOVSKY, 1965; MAYOR and JORDAN, 1966) being consistent with the size of the core as observed in ultrathin sections. Only very few data were presented on the structure and size of the capsomeres surrounding the core. According to BREESE et al. (1964) and GREEN and KARASAKI (1965) they are small morphological units of 2 and 4 nm, respectively, whereas VASQUEZ and BRAILOVSKY (1965) in further characterization suggested them to be rods, 3 nm long and 2 nm wide. In either H-1, RV, X-14, and RT-virus 32 of these capsomeres in $5:3:2$ symmetrical arrangement were proposed to form an icosahedral capsid, a pentakis dodekahedron, with only small gaps and of outstanding stability (BREESE et al., 1964; GREEN and KARASAKI, 1965; VASQUEZ and BRAILOVSKY, 1965; KARASAKI, 1966; MAYOR and JORDAN, 1966; MAYOR and MELNICK, 1966).

3. Physicochemical Properties

a) Type and Configuration of Nucleic Acid

That DNA is incorporated in the hamster-osteolytic viruses as essentiel nucleic acid is well supported by circumstantial observations, indirect methods, and direct isolation of the DNA molecules from purified virus suspensions. Both in vivo and in vitro infection of cells by RV, H-1, H-3, and X-14 virus may result in the formation of basophilic intranuclear inclusion bodies comparable to those frequently associated with the multiplication of well-known DNA-viruses (DAW et al., 1961; BERNHARD et al., 1963; KILHAM and MOLONEY, 1964; FERM and KILHAM, 1964; RUFFALO et al., 1966; MAYOR and JORDAN, 1966). As shown by means of the immunofluorescent technique, these inclusions contain viral antigen and stain Feulgen positive (BERNHARD et al., 1963; HAMPTON, 1964; NICOLETTI et al., 1970). After treatment of infected cell cultures with acridine orange, the inclusion bodies exhibited a brightly green fluorescence consistent with the features of double-stranded DNA. HAMPTON (1964) could not abolish this staining behaviour by previous treatment of the inclusions with DNase and, hence, concluded that the DNA might be contained within virus particles, the protein-coat of which prevented the action of the nuclease. On the contrary, MAYOR and JORDAN (1966) reported the loss of yellow-green staining material from X-14 virus specific inclusion bodies after pre-treatment of cells with DNase.

Further indirect evidence for the DNA-nature of viral nucleic acid has been provided by successful inhibition of virus multiplication by DNA antagonists. PAYNE et al. (1963) found that 5-fluoro-2'-deoxyuridine (FUdR) inhibits replication of X-14 virus in cultures of rat embryonic cells. COCHRAN and PAYNE (1964) confirmed this observation and in addition were able to neutralize the action of FUdR by the simultaneous addition of thymidine to the culture medium. Quite the same results could be obtained for RT-virus (SIEGL et al., unpublished). 5-iodo-2'-deoxyuridine (IUdR) also proved to be effective in reducing the synthesis of complete H-1 virus in "Salk monkey heart" cells (LEDINKO, 1967), while at the same time influencing the formation of H-1 specific hemagglutinin to less an extent.

In parallel to the experiments with IUdR, LEDINKO also tested the inhibitory property of 1-β-D-arabinofuranosylcytosine (ara C) in the same virus/cell system. Added in concentrations of 10—240 µg/ml to the culture media, this DNA-antimetabolite prevented both the synthesis of infectious particles and intracellular accumulation of hemagglutinin, whereas the multiplication of the RNA-containing poliovirus was not affected. Comparable to the possible reversal of the effect of deoxyuridine derivates, ara C-dependent inhibition of H-1 replication finally could be abolished by addition of deoxycytidine.

Attempts to obtain more reliable information on both type and configuration of the nucleic acid enclosed in the hamster-osteolytic viruses were started already in 1965. At that time WHALLEY (1965) noted successful labeling of RV with ^{3}H-thymidine in tissue cultures whereas ^{3}H-uridine was not incorporated. CHEONG and coworkers (1965), estimating the chemical composition of H-1 virus, found 25 per cent of the particle's total mass to be consistent with the features of a double-stranded DNA. The isolated nucleic acid was of an exceptional stability and still proved to be infective for susceptible tissue culture cells after heating to 100° C for 7 minutes. Results apparently also supporting double-stranded configuration of RV-DNA finally were reported by MAY et al. (1967).

Data suggesting the DNA of the hamster-osteolytic viruses to be of single-stranded configuration were obtained for the first time when JAMISON and MAYOR (1965) stained drop preparations of highly concentrated, purified X-14 virus with acridine orange. These authors then observed the typical red fluorescence known to be characteristic for complexes of the dye and RNA or single-stranded DNA. After destruction of the viral capsid by fixation and treatment with pepsin, RNase was ineffective in altering the staining behaviour; digestion with DNase, however, prevented the appearance of any fluorescence. Following closely the methods of MAYOR and DIWAN (1961) and MAYOR and HILL (1961), it could also be shown that purified preparations of RT-virus behaved like X-14 virus during acridine orange staining and, thus, a single-stranded configuration of the DNA likewise must be assumed for this viral agent (SIEGL et al., unpublished). The results of recent physicochemical studies performed with extracted nucleic acid now provided irrefutable evidence for the single-stranded nature of the DNA of both RV and H-1 virus (ROBINSON and HETRICK, 1968; USATEGUI-GOMEZ et al., 1969; MCGEOCH et al., 1970; MAY and MAY, 1970; SALZMANN et al., 1971).

There are three special features of the nucleic acid of both viruses supporting this statement: In contrast to the behaviour of a double-stranded DNA molecule, the isolated nucleic acids during thermal denaturation were found to have a melting profile devoid of a clear cut melting point. They readily reacted with formaldehyde and, subsequent to alkali denaturation and neutralization, banded at the same density in CsCl-gradients as native DNA. From the results presented by the above authors, it also might be concluded that, with regard to further characteristics, the DNA's of RV and H-1 virus are very similar. Either molecule, whether native or alkali-denatured, showed a buoyant density of about 1.72 g/ml in neutral CsCl. Moreover, the DNA of both H-1 and RV apparently sediments at 27 S in neutral solution and at 16.5 S in alkaline solution and based on buoyancy as well as on direct analysis, a base composition consistent with 42 to 45 mole per cent of guanine + cytosine was estimated.

Different opinions exist concerning the molecular weight of the DNA strands. Whereas USATEGUI-GOMEZ et al. (1969) calculated $2.3-3.1 \times 10^6$ daltons for H-1 from their results, McGEOCH and coworkers reported the molecular weight of RV and H-1 DNA to be 1.7×10^6. On the other hand, ROBINSON and HETRICK (1968) starting from the length of RV-DNA (1.30μ) as observable in the electron microscope and applying half the value of 192 daltons/Å of double-stranded DNA, suggested a molecular weight of only 1.2×10^6 daltons. This value, however, will rise to 1.6×10^6 daltons when calculated from strand length on the basis of the same weight per unit length ratio that has been used by CRAWFORD et al. (1969) for the DNA of the minute virus of mice (MVM). It is then also compatible with the finding of SALZMAN et al. (1971) who, by means of electron microscopy and digestion with exonuclease I, showed that the DNA extractable from RV is a single-stranded, linear molecule with a molecular weight of approximately 1.6×10^6 daltons.

b) Structural Proteins

The molecular weight of both RV and H-1 virus has been estimated at 6.6×10^6 daltons (SALZMAN and WHITE, 1970; McGEOCH et al., 1970) of which about 75 per cent or 4.8 to 4.9×10^6 daltons is protein. By dissociation of purified virions and electrophoresis on SDS-polyacrylamide gels this protein could be separated into three components. For RV the molecular weights of the individual proteins were determined to be approximately 72,000, 62,000, and 55,000 daltons (SALZMAN and WHITE, 1970), whereas for H-1 virus figures of 92,000, 72,000, and 56,000 have been reported (KONGSVIK and TOOLAN, 1972). In both viruses the medium-sized component of 62,000 or 72,000 accounted for 75 per cent of total protein mass and, therefore, was suggested to be identical with the capsid protein. There is now strong evidence for the low molecular weight protein to be a contaminant rather than an integral part of the mature virus particle. KONGSVIK and coworkers (1974) have reanalysed the polypeptide composition of H-1 virus isolated from synchronized NB-cell cultures and, in contrast to previous findings, only could demonstrate a major component of 72,000 and a minor one with 92,000 daltons.

The significance of the minor polypeptide as well as of the third protein is not known. It may be discussed, however, whether one of them might be associated with a DNA polymerase activity. SALZMAN (1971) was able to show such an enzymatic activity cosedimenting with RV virions purified by at least two density equilibrium centrifugations in CsCl. Yet, attempts to repeat these experiments and to characterize a similar polymerase activity in association with H-1 virus failed (RHODE, 1974a).

c) Buoyant Density and Sedimentation Behaviour

Buoyant density studies in CsCl revealed tissue culture harvests of RV and H-1 viruses to be composed of particles with different properties. During gradient centrifugation the virus suspensions regularly separate into two main bands, a heavy one consisting of almost exclusively complete hemagglutinating and fully infective virus particles and a light one of low infectivity but containing large amounts of hemagglutinating particle fragments and empty capsids. Whereas all investigators in conformity reported the density of the light band to be 1.30 to 1.32 g/ml in CsCl (e.g. JAMISON and MAYOR, 1965; WHALLEY, 1965; GREEN and KARASAKI, 1965; USATEGUI-GOMEZ et al., 1969; MAY and MAY, 1970), extreme values of 1.37 and 1.47 g/ml were measured for the complete particles (EL DADAH et al., 1967; McGEOCH et al., 1970). Most frequently, however, figures around 1.40 g/ml have been noted and at the present time it is not possible to decide whether RV, X-14, H-1, as well as the HER-agent may be distinguished on the basis of their buoyancy (BREESE et al., 1964; VASQUEZ and BRAILOVSKY, 1965; WHALLEY, 1965; PAYNE et al., 1964; COCHRAN and PAYNE, 1964; CHEONG et al., 1965; ROBINSON and HETRICK, 1968). Finally, it should be mentioned that RV —apparently due to a different solvation of the particles—accumulated in potassium tartrate gradients at densities around 1.31—1.32 g/ml (WHITMAN and HETRICK, 1967; BREESE et al., 1964; WHALLEY, 1965).

Fractionation of the gradients, in addition to the two main bands, occasionally revealed distinct accumulation of virus particles in further density zones. Thus, at an intermediate density of 1.38 g/ml ROBINSON and HETRICK (1968) noted an additional peak for rat virus, which—according to electron microscopic examination—proved to be composed of "full" and "empty" viral particles. Since such a peak also appeared after recentrifugation of the isolated heavy virus band, the authors suggested the particles to be only breakdown products of the complete virions. Working with the same virus, E. MAY and P. MAY (1970) even observed two more small bands. Whereas the one with a mean density of 1.37 g/ml is consistent with the observation of ROBINSON and HETRICK, there is so far no information concerning the significance of those virus particles found at a density range of 1.45—1.47 g/ml.

The sedimentation coefficients of both RV and H-1 virus were determined by McGEOCH et al. (1970). With a $S_{20,w}$ of 110 ± 2, these viruses sediment at the same rate as MVM (CRAWFORD et al., 1969) and at a rate very similar to phage ΦX 174 ($S_{20,w} = 112$, CRAWFORD et al., 1969) as well as to parvoviruses isolated by HALLAUER and KRONAUER (1962) (105 ± 12; SIEGL et al., 1971) (see Table 7, p. 87).

d) Resistance to Physical and Chemical Agents

The resistance of the hamster-osteolytic agents to physical and chemical treatment has been investigated using virus suspensions of varying purity. Frequently the test methods were applied to crude tissue culture harvests or filtrates of homogenates of organs exstirpated from animals dead from virus infection. Only in very few cases purified virus samples were tested. Although the results, therefore, provide no identical basis for evaluation, they nevertheless suggest the hamster-osteolytic agents to be grouped within the most stable viruses so far known.

(1) *Heat- and pH-Stability*

KILHAM and OLIVIER (1959) heated RV in tissue culture fluids for 2 hours to 80° C and noted no loss of infectivity. In a quite similar experiment using however a suspension of RV in culture medium to which 10 per cent calf serum had been added, BRAILOVSKY (1966), on the other hand, recorded a decline of the infective titer from 10^6 to 10^4 PFU/ml. Comparable results were also obtained for the antigenically related LS-virus. Treatment of this agent for 1 hour at 75° C resulted in a 90 per cent loss and at 85° C in a complete loss of the infective potency (LUM and SCHREINER, 1963).

In parallel to the decrease of the infective titer, the hemagglutinating activity of the RV-sample used by BRAILOVSKY was reduced from 512 to 16 hemagglutinating units (HAU) after 2 hours at 80° C. Moreover, data presented by GREEN (1965) and SIEGL et al. (1971) showed that the stability of the hemagglutinins of RV, H-1, H-3, X-14, and RT-virus at elevated temperatures in addition depends on the pH of the suspension medium. According to GREEN, the hemagglutinin of H-1 virus proved to be relatively stable from pH 2 through pH 11 when the virus was held at 4°, 25°, and 37° C for 30 minutes. With rising temperature a gradual fall of HA-titer occurred especially at extreme pH values. In virus suspensions held at pH 5 and 6, however, active hemagglutinin still could be demonstrated after 30 minutes at 80° C. These observations on H-1 stability were confirmed by SIEGL and coworkers. In addition, experiments with RV, H-3, X-14, and RT-virus conducted in parallel demonstrated the exceptional uniform behaviour of the hemagglutinin of the various virus particles. There was only one obvious difference between H-1 and RTV, as well as the viruses serologically related to RV. Whereas the latter agents were stable at 56° C throughout the whole pH range tested, the hemagglutinin titers of H-1 at that temperature had already decreased in solutions of pH 2 and pH 11.

(2) *UV-Irradiation and Ultrasonication*

At room temperature, RV and H-1 virus were found to be readily inactivated by UV-light (KILHAM and OLIVIER, 1959; TOOLAN et al., 1960). On the other hand, ultrasonication will not affect the infectivity of the virus particles as long as too extented a treatment does not result in an undue heating of the virus suspensions. BRAILOVSKY (1966) sonicated suspensions of RV in cell culture medium at 10^6 cycles per second and observed neither a decline in infectivity nor a change in hemagglutination titer during a period of 16 minutes. Therefore, ultrasonication successfully may be used to liberate intracellular virus from infected cells (BREESE et al., 1964; VASQUEZ and BRAILOVSKY, 1965).

(3) *Organic Solvents*

Both infectivity and the hemagglutinating property of the hamster-osteolytic agents are not affected by treatment with ether (KILHAM and OLIVIER, 1959; LUM and SCHREINER, 1963; GREEN, 1964; EL DADAH et al., 1967), chloroform (SIEGL et al., 1971) or various alcohols (GREEN, 1964). Moreover, according to BREESE et al. (1964) and GREEN and KARASAKI (1965), shaking of virus suspensions with butanol provides an useful means of obtaining pure virus samples.

(4) *Enzymes*

Special investigations concerning the resistance of the virus particles to enzyme digestion were reported by GREEN (1964) as well as by KONGSVIK and TOOLAN (1972) for H-1, H-3, and RV. Neither RNase and DNase, nor trypsin, chymotrypsin, and papain had any effect on infectivity or hemagglutinating activity. Therefore, the enzymes listed above were oftenly used (VASQUEZ and BRAILOVSKY, 1965; TOOLAN *et al.*, 1967; MAY and MAY, 1970) to purify tissue culture harvests of H-1 and RV from cellular nucleic acids and proteins.

(5) *Storage*

In accordance to the low effect of heat on their biologic activities, the viruses were found to survive storage at proper conditions for a very long time without any undue loss of infectivity. H-1, HB, HT, and H-3 virus prepared as distilled water filtrates of infected hamster livers were kept under refrigeration for more than 6 years and were then still fully infective (TOOLAN *et al.*, 1960; GREEN, 1964; GREEN and KARASAKI, 1965; TOOLAN, 1968). The preservation of RV has not been tested during a comparable space of time, yet, KILHAM and OLIVIER (1959) observed no reduction in titer when storing the virus at $-40°$ C for six months and WHITMAN and HETRICK (1967) noted that purified RV suspended either in 10^{-3} M EDTA or medium 199 readily survived at temperatures from $+4°$ to $-60°$ C for as long as 60 days. At room temperature, however, LUM and SCHREINER (1963) found the infectivity of LS-virus to decline by almost 99 per cent within three weeks. More than 90 per cent of infectivity was lost after lyophilization and subsequent storage at $-20°$ C for a period of three months.

4. Antigenic Structure and Serologic Relationship

Injection of the hamster-osteolytic viruses into animals induces the formation of neutralizing, hemagglutination-inhibiting, as well as complement-fixing antibodies. The site of the corresponding antigen(s) within the virion is unknown, but HA and N antigens can be assumed to be located at the surface of the particle. Moreover, results obtained by means of gradient centrifugation, hemagglutination, and biochemical studies (PAYNE *et al.*, 1964; GREEN and KARASAKI, 1965; CASTRO *et al.*, 1971) suggested the hemagglutinating antigen to be a protein devoid of lipids and glycoids.

a) *Hemagglutinin and Hemagglutination*

The ability to agglutinate erythrocytes of different species is one of the most outstanding features of the hamster-osteolytic viruses. This property already has been recognized by KILHAM and OLIVIER (1959) with RV and since then has provided the simplest method of demonstrating the presence of the viruses. However, independent of whether organ tissues of infected animals or tissue cultures served as a source for isolation, the hemagglutinin proved to be highly cell-associated. Optimum amounts of hemagglutinin and, at the same time, of infectious virus, therefore could be obtained only after dissociation of the virus from cell debris by means of treatment with deoxycholate, RDE, or, most effectively, by the alkaline extraction method introduced by HALLAUER and

KRONAUER (1962). The latter technique provides the additional possibility to test for the presence of parvoviruses in tissue cultures without destroying the cell monolayer.

The ability to agglutinate red blood cells is the characteristic of mature virions, incomplete particles, and empty capsids. The infectivity/HA ratio therefore varies considerably depending on the degree to which infectious virions have been freed from incomplete particles. For crude tissue culture harvests of H-1 and of X-14 virus MOORE (1962) and PAYNE (1964) have reported that 10^3—10^4 $TCID_{50}$ were necessary to give a positive hemagglutination at a dilution of 1 in 80. Smaller figures, however, are usually obtained following the extraction of hemagglutinin from tissue cultures by Hallauer's method. The alkaline buffer liberates virus particles from cell debris, and, by some unknown mechanism, releases hemagglutinating capsid structures from infected but so far undestroyed cells.

The interaction between the hemagglutinin of the hamster-osteolytic agents and erythrocytes of various species was shown to be quite a stable one. Agglutination takes place at $4°$ C, room temperature, as well as at $37°$ C (TOOLAN, 1968; HALLAUER et al., 1971) and no spontaneous elution occurs at room temperature. Treatment with receptor destroying enzyme (RDE), however, results in a complete dissociation of the formed virus/red blood cell complex (PAYNE et al., 1964). Furthermore, pretreatment of erythrocytes with either the —LEE strain of influenza virus (MOORE, 1962), lipid solvents, or periodate—but not with formaldehyde or trypsin—completely destroyed the cell receptors for the hemagglutinins of RV, H-1, and X-14 viruses. The respective receptors, therefore, were proposed to be a glycolipid containing N-acetyl-neuraminic acid linked with carbohydrates and fatty acids (COCUZZA and RUSSO, 1969).

Table 2 summarizes the observations on the hemagglutination spectrum of the hamster-osteolytic agents. Every positive agglutination of red blood cells of a certain species has been included though some of the results could not be corroborated. All data, however, are in good accordance concerning the affinity of the viruses for red blood cells of guinea pig origin. With exception of HT-virus, they also agglutinate rat erythrocytes. The suitability of human erythrocytes for hemagglutination tests, however, is still a matter of discussion. It is accepted for H-1 virus and RTV and, probably, may be taken for sure in the case of H-3.

On several occasions it was proposed that the particular isolates of the hamster-osteolytic viruses might be distinguished on the basis of their specific hemagglutination pattern. In this respect reliable conclusions however can only be obtained under standardized test conditions. Experiments fullfilling this prerequisite have been reported by TOOLAN (1967) and by HALLAUER et al. (1972). These authors postulated a similar hemagglutination titer of all viruses with guinea pig erythrocytes as the prerequisite for standardization. Moreover, only one single batch of a certain red blood cell was used throughout the experiment. The results thus obtained form the backbone of Table 8 (p. 88) in which the hemagglutination spectra of all viruses belonging to the genus Parvovirus are summarized. They clearly demonstrate that the possibility to distinguish strains of one and the same serotype on the basis of the respective hemagglutination pattern is limited. Obvious and reliable differences have been noted only for H-1 virus and the serologically related HT isolate (TOOLAN, 1967): H-1 preferentially agglutinated

Table 2. Red Blood Cells Agglutinated by Strains of the "Hamster-Osteolytic" Viruses

Virus	Human	Monkey	Guinea pig	Rat	Hamster	Mouse	Gerbil	Rabbit	Agouti	Sheep	Goat	Horse	Cattle	Pig	Cat	Dog	Chicken	Goose	Duck	Frog	References
RV	+	+	+	+	+	+	−	−	+	+		+	−	+	+	+	+	−	+		82, 131, 180, 197, 200, 256
H-3	+	+	+	+	+	+	−	+	+	+	−	+	−	+	+	+	+	+	+	+	82, 180, 200, 256
X-14	+	−	+	+	+	+		+		+		+	−	+	+	+	+	−		−	82, 97, 198
HER	−	−	+							−											52
RTV	+	+	+	+	+	+		−		+		+	−	+	+	+	+	+			82
H-1	+	+	+	+	+	+	+	−	+	+		+	−	+	+	+	+	+	+	+	82, 180, 200, 256
HT	−	−	+	−	+	−	−	−	+	−		−			+	+	−	−	+		256
HB	−	−	+	+	+	+	−	−	−	−		−			−	−	−	−	+		256

Origin of red blood cells

guinea pig red blood cells and, in a diminishing degree, erythrocytes of hamster, human, and rat origin. HT-virus, on the other hand, showed a similar affinity for guinea pig and hamster erythrocytes but agglutinated neither human nor rat red blood cells.

Closely related to their hemagglutination property, the phenomenon of hemadsorption associated with the hamster-osteolytic viruses shall be recorded lastly. PORTELLA (1963) successfully used this phenomenon to select infected cells from monolayers for ultrahistological investigations. He was able to show that in tissue cultures infected with either RV, H-1, or H-3 virus, only those cells to which guinea pig erythrocytes were attached both as single or clumps of cells contained demonstrable virus particles. As evident from electron micrographs, attachment of the red blood cells took place under the direct participation of virus particles which served as the connecting link between the cytoplasmic membrane of the cultured cell and the surface of the erythrocyte. PORTELLA recommended hemadsorption especially for infectivity endpoint titrations, since positive reactions usually can be recorded as early as three days after infection, i.e. usually before the appearance of cytopathic changes.

b) Hemagglutination Inhibition

Inhibition of hemagglutination by means of specific homologous as well as heterologous antisera presented an easy and quick method to reveal the antigenic relationship between the hemagglutinins of the hamster-osteolytic agents. Thereby, H-1 and HT-virus on the one hand and RV, H-3, X-14, LS, and HER-virus on the other, were found to share a common antigen (compare Table 9, p. 90) whereas HB as well as RT virus proved to be completely unrelated (MOORE, 1962; PORTELLA, 1964; PAYNE et al., 1963; LUM and SCHREINER, 1963; TOOLAN, 1964; TOOLAN and LEDINKO, 1965; EL DADAH et al., 1967; HALLAUER et al., 1971). In addition, only an insignificant reciprocal antigenic relationship of any of these viruses with other parvoviruses was observed (e.g. HALLAUER et al., 1971).

The significance of HI-experiments may be influenced by nonspecific inhibitors present in both normal and immune-sera of rats, hamsters, rabbits, cattle, and man (MOORE, 1962; LUM, 1970; HALLAUER et al., 1972). Attempts to remove the inhibitor by means of treating the sera with RDE, trypsin, or sodium periodate were unsuccessful. Extraction of sera with kaolin according to CLARKE and CASALS (1958), on the contrary, resulted in serum samples almost free of inhibitory effect and reduced the antibody titer only to a limited extent.

An outstanding hemagglutination inhibiting substance has been isolated by TOOLAN (1964) from the placenta of a two months ectopic pregnancy and, later on, from all human placentas tested. The inhibitor almost specifically interfered with the hemagglutination by H-1 virus, whereas the hemagglutinins of HT and HB-viruses were only occasionally and those of RV and H-3 virus were never inhibited. Since the inhibitor could be isolated neither from maternal or fetal sera nor from urine or amniotic fluids, TOOLAN (1968) assumed the substance to be a specific product of the placenta.

In the isolated and purified state the inhibitor proved to be rather resistant to changes in temperature and pH. No loss of activity was recorded after heating to 100° C for 60 minutes or by varying the pH between 1 and 9. Its activity was destroyed, however, by treatment with trypsin, chymotrypsin, papain, neuraminidase, and sodium periodate. Together with additional observations on electrophoretic mobility and sedimentation behaviour, these data suggested the substance to be a glycoprotein with properties of a macroglobulin (USATEGUI-GOMEZ, 1965; USATEGUI-GOMEZ and MORGAN, 1968). It is especially worthwhile to mention the exceptional high specifity of the purified inhibitor for H-1 hemagglutinin which is still inhibited by concentrations as low as 0.004 μg/ml, whereas the hemagglutination induced by RV and H-3 viruses is not influenced even by the undiluted inhibitor.

c) Cross Neutralization

Neutralization tests performed both in newborn hamsters and in tissue cultures reflected the very same antigenic grouping of the hamster-osteolytic viruses as recorded from hemagglutination inhibiton experiments. Neutralizing antibodies to H-1 or HT virus were of similar efficiency in reducing the infectivity of either agent but did not interfere with multiplication of HB, RV, and H-3 virus (TOOLAN, 1964, 1968). HB virus again proved to be unrelated to other agents (TOOLAN, 1964) and homologous as well as heterologous antibodies to RV, H-3, and LS virus neutralized infectivity of the respective viruses to a similar extent (MOORE, 1962; PORTELLA, 1963; LUM and SCHREINER, 1963). Nevertheless, serologic differences between the members of an antigenic group could be recorded occasionally. Their significance shall be discussed in section 4e).

d) Complement Fixation and Immunofluorescent Studies

CROSS and PARKER (1972) have analysed the antigenic relationship of RV, H-1, and of the minute virus of mice (MVM) by complement fixation and immunofluorescent studies conducted in parallel with hemagglutination and neutralization tests. Whereas complement fixation, in agreement with the results of hemagglutination inhibition and neutralization, showed the three viruses to be of distinct antigenicity, immunofluorescent staining suggested some common antigen to be present in both RV and H-1 virus infected rat embryo cells. The antisera used for staining of infected cultures had been produced by injection of cell-free but otherwise unpurified tissue culture harvests of the viruses. Therefore, it remains unclear whether the antigen in common is really included in the mature virion, whether it is a replication related protein coded for by the nucleic acid of RV as well as of H-1 virus, or whether it is merely a contaminating host cell protein.

e) Differences in Antigenic Composition between Various Virus Strains

Studies concerning the antigenic relationship of the different agents (see sections 4b, and 4c) revealed that all strains could be grouped into four distinct classes. The results were the same whether obtained by cross neutralization or hemagglutination-inhibition tests and most of the isolated viruses—H-3, LS, X-14, Krisini, and the HER-agent—were shown to be closely related to RV. H-1 is the prototype virus of a further serologic class, into which so far only HT has been included as a second member. HB-virus as well as RT-virus, finally, seem to be unrelated to all the other virus strains.

MOORE (1962), PORTELLA (1963), and LUM and SCHREINER (1964) noticed that, although there was cross-neutralization between RV and H-3, or RV and LS-virus, respectively, the immune sera showed considerably higher titer for the homologous than for the heterologous virus. LUM and SCHREINER even reported an 8 to 128 times elevated neutralizing capacity for the homologous antisera. Moreover, hyperimmune serum obtained after repeated injections of H-3 virus also inhibited the hemagglutination properties of H-1 virus, an effect not observed with ordinary immune sera. As there is no evidence that the H-3 virus stock used for inoculation had been examined for a possible contamination with H-1, the latter observation is not very conclusive. The results obtained with RV, H-3, and LS-virus, however, may really account for some differences in antigenicity.

The data presented by NICHOLSON and HETRICK (1969) regarding host influence on the antigenic composition of RV might be looked upon as providing a possible basis for evaluation of such an antigenic difference. Repeated passage of this virus in either rat embryo cell cultures or in suckling hamsters was reported to result in two different virus strains, the protein coat of which could be distinguished by electrophoretic analysis, neutralization, and HI-tests. These alterations proved to be reversible after mere changing of the culture system and, therefore, apparently were host-controlled. The possibility that host proteins were incorporated into the virus capsids can only be considered valid as long as these antigens were altered in structure during incorporation and, hence, could be no longer recognized by antibodies to normal host tissue material.

5. Cultivation

a) Host-Cell Range

In spite of the observations that latent RV- and H-1 virus infections are present in laboratory rats at a high incidence and that the virus may be transmitted vertically to the progeny (e.g. MOORE and NICASTRI, 1965; ROBEY et al., 1968; KILHAM and MARGOLIS, 1969) primary and secondary cultures of embryonic rat cells were frequently preferred for in vitro cultivation of hamster-osteolytic viruses. Primary cultures of embryonic cells of human, chicken, calf, and mouse origin proved to be unsuitable and in cultures of embryonic hamster cells the replication of RV, H-1, and H-3 was found to be only accompanied by slowly progressive CPE. The cultural behaviour of the particular hamster-osteolytic viruses is summarized in Table 3.

To exclude the undesired presence of latent RV and H-1 infections in tissue culture cells, permanent rat cell lines controlled for many passages were supposed to provide an excellent and virus-free culture system. In two instances, however, high passages of either the rat nephroma cell line established by BABCOCK and SOUTHAM (1967) or the AT cell line of Tournier were shown to harbour RV (WOZNIAK and HETRICK, 1969) and RTV (HALLAUER et al., 1971), respectively. Attempts to use cell lines derived from tissues of other species confirmed the narrow host cell range of some hamster-osteolytic viruses (Table 4). Thus, X-14 and RT-virus multiplied only in permanent rat cell cultures, while RV could be regularly grown both in rat cell strains and in stable lines of hamster kidney cells. From the investigations of LUM and SCHREINER (1963) there was also some indication

Table 3. *Host-Cell Spectrum of Strains of the "Hamster-Osteolytic" Viruses in Primary Cell Cultures*

Origin and type of cells	Virus						References
	RV	H-3	X-14	HER	LS	H-1	
Rat, embryonic	+	+	+	+	+	+	52, 131, 154, 180, 190, 197
Hamster, embryonic	+	+				+	116, 180
Mouse, embryonic	—	—	—		—	—	131, 154, 180, 197
Bovine, embryonic	—				—		154
Chicken, embryonic	—		—		—		154, 191
Human, embryonic	—	—	—			—	180
embryonic kidney	—					—	260
amnion	—	—				—	260

that the human amniotic cell line FL might be susceptible for RV as well as for the serologically related LS-agent. For H-1 and H-3 virus, on the other hand, the spectrum of susceptible cell lines comprised those of human, monkey, rat, and hamster origin.

b) Cytopathogenicity

With only very few exceptions multiplication of the hamster-osteolytic agents in tissue cultures usually provokes a cytopathic effect which is demonstrable both by mere microscopic observation of unstained cell sheets and by means of histologic staining methods. According to the observations of KILHAM and OLIVIER (1959), MOORE (1962), and TOOLAN and LEDINKO (1965), the CPE is initiated by granulation of the infected cells followed by their rounding up, and finally, by detachment of necrotic cells from the destroyed monolayer. Histologic staining of infected tissue cultures in addition revealed some virus-dependent cell alterations consisting largely in the formation of intranuclear inclusion bodies. In all cultures susceptible for infection these inclusions could be readily demonstrated by means of H & E, Giemsa, methyl pyronine, acridine orange, or Feulgen staining (DAWE et al., 1961; MOORE, 1962; BERNHARD et al., 1963; HAMPTON, 1964; MAYOR and JORDAN, 1966; NICOLETTI et al., 1969). In accordance with the ob-

Table 4. *Host-Cell Spectrum of Strains of the "Hamster-Osteolytic" Viruses in Permanent Cell Lines*

Origin and name of cell line	Virus						References
	RV	H-3	X-14	LS	RTV	H-1	
Rat:							
AT (Tournier)	+	+	+		+	+	15, 82
Rat nephroma	+						209
(Babcock & Southam)							
Hamster:							
BHK	+					+	15
BHK 21	+	+	−		−	+	82
BHK 35	+	+	−		−	+	82
HaK (Spense)		+				+	260
Mouse:							
L 929	−			−			154
L (?)	−	−	−		−	−	82
Human:							
HeLa	−	+	−		−	+	82, 260
HeLa S-3		+				+	260
KB	−	+	−		−	+	82
HEp-2	−	+	−		−	+	82
FL amnion	−	+	−		−	+	82, 260
AV-3 amnion	−			−			154
Liver (Chang)		+				+	260
Intestine (Henle)		+				+	260
Conjunctiva (Chang)		+				+	260
NB embryonic kidney		+				+	260
(Shein & Enders)							
"monkey heart" (Salk)		+				+	260
Monkey:							
Rhesus kidney,		−				−	260
LLC-MK-2 (Hull)							
Chimpanzee liver		+				+	260
(Douglas)							
Vero	−	−	−		−	−	82

servations of NICOLETTI *et al.* (1969) on multiplication of RV, X-14, and H-1 virus, BERNHARD *et al.* (1963) noted that the first signs of RV infection in susceptible cells occurred as early as 36—48 hours post infection. At that time single cells of the monolayers already showed evidence for margination of nuclear chromatin, the appearance of isolated or multiple granules, or even dense homogenous masses stained Feulgen-positive and, after acridine orange treatment, exhibited a bright yellowish-green fluorescence. Moreover, the inclusion bodies also could be demonstrated by use of specific fluorescein-conjugated antibodies and, hence, proved to be accumulations of virus-specific antigens (HAMPTON, 1964; MAYOR and ITO, 1968; COLE and NATHANSON, 1969).

It should be mentioned that after cytochemical studies on rat embryonic cell cultures infected by either RV, H-1, or H-3 virus, HAMPTON (1964) and MOORE and NICASTRI (1965) reported differences in the intranuclear changes produced by the particular agents. The significance of these observations, however, is unknown.

With regard to rapidity of appearance, progress, and severity the CPE depends on several essential factors. First of all, the time necessary for development of a clear cut CPE in confluent monolayers of fully susceptible cells was found to be directly related to the amount of virus inoculated. High inoculation doses of RV, H-1, H-3, and LS-virus resulted in cytopathic changes as early as 4 to 6 days post inoculation, whereas with endpoint dilutions of virus samples a CPE could only be detected after an observation time of 19 to 21 days (MOORE, 1962; LUM and SCHREINER, 1963; TOOLAN and LEDINKO, 1965). Second, as replication of the viruses is controlled by cellular physiology, progress of virus multiplication and, at the same time, progress of CPE is favoured by an elevated mitotic activity of the cultured cells. Finally, a third limiting factor consists in the extent to which a virus has been adapted to a particular type of cells. A potent experiment to exemplify this has been reported by TOOLAN and LEDINKO (1965). Studying the multiplication of H-1 and H-3 virus in permanent cell lines of human, monkey, and hamster origin as well as in secondary cultures of hamster embryonic cells, TOOLAN and LEDINKO noted that, despite of the apparently similar progress of virus multiplication in all cell types tested, there was initially a clear cut difference in the cytopathic response of the culture systems to infection with either agent. For both H-1 and H-3 virus maximum hemagglutinin titers could be demonstrated 3 to 4 days after infection. However, only for the well adapted H-1 virus maximum virus synthesis also was paralleled by cytopathic changes. The CPE induced by H-3 virus on the contrary, was of retarded appearance and showed a much slower progress. Nevertheless, it finally reached the same degree as the CPE produced by H-1 virus. After 3 to 5 successive tissue culture passages of H-3 virus, however, its replication became indistinguishable from the behaviour of H-1 virus both in regard to the synchronous appearance of maximum hemagglutinin titers and CPE and to the progress of the cytopathic changes.

c) Plaque Formation

In tissue cultures infected with endpoint dilutions of the hamster-osteolytic viruses the development of virus-specific cellular changes is frequently obscured by age-dependent degeneration of the cell sheet during the long observation period necessary. BRAILOVSKY (1966) and LEDINKO (1967) tried to overcome these difficulties by plaque titration for RV and H-1 virus, respectively.

BRAILOVSKY used confluent monolayers of rat embryonic cells. The relationship between the number of plaques and the virus dilutions inoculated proved to be linear only when the inoculum was allowed to adsorb to the cells for at least 2 hours. Moreover, staining of the monolayers with neutral red earlier than 72 hours post infection frequently reduced the plaque yield. Under constant conditions RV specific, distinct plaques 3—4 mm in size already could be counted five days after inoculation. With longer incubation time they still increased in diameter, yet, their number remained constant.

Plaque titration of H-1 virus in monolayers of Salk-monkey-heart cells (these cells were shown to be of human origin) brought about no significant advantage in contrast to titration of infectivity by the culture tube technique. The virus induced distinct CPE in normal tissue cultures already 4—6 days following infection (TOOLAN and LEDINKO, 1965). However, only 90 per cent of small, 1.7 ± 1.2 mm sized plaques were present 12 days p.i. when techniques quite similar to those of BRAILOVSKY were applied. Additional plaques appeared very slowly and final reading of titers could only be done 16 days post inoculation.

d) Virus Multiplication

Data concerning the intracellular multiplication of the hamster-osteolytic viruses are quite contradictory. Whereas several studies dealing with the multiplication behaviour of H-1, H-3, RV, and X-14 virus suggested virus replication to occur very slowly and to extend for at least 47 hours (MOORE, 1962; HAMPTON, 1964; PAYNE et al., 1964; MAYOR and ITO, 1968; AL LAMI et al., 1969; FONG et al., 1970), other investigations revealed a relatively short growth cycle of only 20—24 hours length (BRAILOVSKY, 1966; COLE and NATHANSON, 1969; RHODE, 1973). Moreover, the various reports are not in accordance whether the exclusive site of virus replication is the nucleus of an infected cell or whether both nucleus and cytoplasm are involved. BRAILOVSKY (1966) and COLE and NATHANSON (1969) claimed that many of the divergent results might be due to insufficient experimental conditions, e.g. the use of cell cultures infected at too low a multiplicity and/or insensitive methods to follow virus growth. This statement could explain some of the observed differences. However, there is now convincing evidence that factors such as the susceptibility of the cells and especially the physiologic state of the tissue cultures at the time of infection play a much more important role.

(1) Growth Cycle in Fully Susceptible Cells

According to COLE and NATHANSON (1969) detectable synthesis of RV in fully susceptible rat embryonic tissue cultures starts in the cytoplasm of an infected cell after a latent period of 5—6 hours. By means of immunofluorescent staining viral antigen then could be already detected in the perinuclear region. Three hours later and lasting about 14 hours p.i. increasing appearance of nuclear and concomitant disappearance of cytoplasmic fluorescence indicated transfer of the antigen across the nuclear membrane. Subsequently, the nuclei—with the exception of the nucleoli—frequently appeared completely filled with viral antigen. Almost 80 per cent of them, however, disappeared at 20 hours p.i. simultaneously with a rapid increase of cell-free virus in the supernatant medium. Accumulation of RV in the nuclei was paralleled by retraction of cytoplasm, pyknosis and, finally, cellular death.

Replication of H-1 virus, on the contrary, has been frequently reported to be characterized by an eclipse period of approximately 10 hours and an overall length of 48—50 hours (HAMPTON, 1964; AL LAMI et al., 1969; FONG et al., 1970). According to more recent results, such a growth cycle is only representative for the accumulation of progeny virus in a culture system based on randomly growing cells. RHODE (1973) provided evidence that multiplication of H-1 virus depends strongly on the cellular events in late S-phase of the infected cell and, if viral replication is followed in a parasynchronous cell system, the growth cycle parameters are comparable to those of RV.

At the ultrastructural level, there was evidence especially for those steps of the multiplication of RV, H-1, and X-14 virus involving intranuclear changes (BERNHARD et al., 1963; PORTELLA, 1964; MAYOR and JORDAN, 1966; AL LAMI et al., 1969). In contrast to the early observations for H-1 virus by CHANDRA and TOOLAN (1961) which claimed an intracytoplasmic and even an intramitochondrial type of replication, first signs of virus multiplication usually were found to consist in a margination of nuclear chromatin and in a condensation of cytoplasm.

At the same time spherical or elongated particles with a diameter of 12—18 nm representing the dark staining core of the hamster-osteolytic agents could be already demonstrated within the nucleus. Later on, large amounts of the virus particles spread throughout the nucleus and sometimes formed loose, but never crystal-like aggregates. At that stage of virus multiplication the first radical changes in nuclear morphology became evident. Frequently splitting of the nuclear membrane could be observed with the inner leaflet deeply invaginating the nucleus. After subsequent disruption of the nuclear membrane the virus particles spread from the disintegrated nucleus to the likewise damaged cytoplasm. Occasionally the virions were found to be embedded in matrix-like elements and vesicles or to be associated with the endoplasmic reticulum and other membrane fragments.

There is one additional observation deserving special discussion. By means of acridine orange staining NICOLETTI et al. (1969) presented evidence for the involvement of the nucleolus during later stages of RV, H-1, and X-14 virus replication. Ultrahistological studies on H-1 virus-infected NB (newborn human kidney cells transformed by SV 40-virus) and SMH (Salk "monkey heart") cells now seem to confirm this observation (AL LAMI et al., 1969). In parallel with the scattering of newly synthesized virus particles all over the nucleus, the nucleoli were found to condense and finally formed doughnut-shaped "nucleolar inclusions" containing empty virus capsids. Due to the fact that the nucleolus apparently was the preferential site for accumulation of virus capsids, AL LAMI and coworkers therefore suggested this organelle to play an important role in H-1 virus synthesis.

(2) Incomplete Growth Cycle

It has been repeatedly noted that although inoculation of RV or H-1 virus into certain types of cells produced a CPE, no viral yields beyond those attributable to input virus finally could be recovered from these culture systems. For H-1 virus such an abortive multiplication behaviour has been reported to occur in cultures of the diploid cell line WI-26 where infection causes the formation of capsid proteins without the production of infective virus. This was also observed to occur in secondary cultures of human embryonic lung cells (LEDINKO and TOOLAN, 1968; LEDINKO et al., 1969). Replication of RV, on the other hand, was only scarcely supported by BHK-21 and L-cells. Immunofluorescent data (COLE and NATHANSON, 1969) suggest that, at least in the latter virus/cell systems, the first steps in virus multiplication might be analogous to those of virus synthesis in fully susceptible cells. Viral antigen, though at a lower intensity, could be demonstrated within the cytoplasm 5 hours post inoculation. In contrast to a complete growth cycle, however, this antigen persisted at an almost constant level and successful viral replication as shown by intranuclear accumulation of fluorescent material was noted only in a few cells.

There is evidence that factors known to favour virus replication in fully susceptible cells—e.g. coinfection with a "helper" adenovirus or an elevated mitotic activity of cells—may successfully convert abortive virus infection into a reproductive one.

(3) Stimulation of Virus Multiplication by "Helper" Viruses

Stimulation of RV and H-1 virus replication using adenovirus type 12 as a "helper" has been reported at two different occasions. BRAILOVSKY and CHANY (1965) noted that synchronous inoculation of the helper virus with either partially UV-inactivated or untreated RV into rat embryonic culture cells led—in contrast to mere RV infection—to a much more rapid formation of a RV-specific CPE as well as a significant rise in recoverable amounts of hemagglutinin and infectious virus. The enhancement of virus multiplication proved to be a linear function of the adenovirus type 12 doses applied (CHANY and BRAILOVSKY, 1965). A similar effect could be obtained when the adenovirus inoculum was replaced by virus-free extracts of tissue cultures previously infected by adenovirus type 12, whilst extracts of uninfected cultures were ineffective. The authors finally attributed the enhancement of RV replication to a stimulating factor ("stimulon") they thought to be coded within the adenovirus genome and synthesized during early stages of the virus multiplication cycle. The activity of this "stimulon" could be destroyed by treatment with trypsin, whereas it was unaffected by DNase and RNase.

LEDINKO and TOOLAN (1968), in addition, reported successful stimulation of H-1 virus replication in secondary cultures of human embryonic lung cells and in monolayers of the human diploid cell line WI-26. Whereas inoculation of these cells with H-1 virus alone resulted in a CPE but never in progressive virus growth, the simultaneous infection with adenovirus type 12 increased the amount of demonstrable H-1 virus within 5 to 6 days to a hundred-fold of the dose inoculated. The effect was absent when the adenovirus was inactivated by UV-light previous to inoculation and—in contrast to the findings of BRAILOVSKY and CHANY (1965)—also after application of virus-free extracts of adenovirus infected cell cultures. Moreover, replication of H-1 virus interfered with the multiplication of the "helper"-adenovirus. It could also be shown that the step rendering cells competent to synthesize H-1 virus apparently occurs late in the adenovirus replicative cycle (LEDINKO et al., 1969). On the other hand, attempts to increase the yield of X-14 virus in rat embryonic cell cultures by additional inoculation of adenovirus type 2 were unsuccessful (MAYOR and JORDAN, 1966).

(4) *Dependence of Virus Multiplication on Cell Physiologic State*

The pronounced destructive action of the hamster-osteolytic viruses in rapidly proliferating tissues after inoculation into newborn hamsters and rats suggested the multiplication of these viruses to be especially favoured by cells in mitosis (MARGOLIS and KILHAM, 1965). Additional evidence supporting this hypothesis has been presented by COLE and NATHANSON (1969) and LEDINKO et al. (1969) who found that the abortive multiplication of RV and H-1 virus in L-cells and cultures of the WI-26 diploid cell line, respectively, was overcome in a small proportion of cells obviously undergoing active growth.

According to the results of more recent studies (TENNANT et al., 1969; HAMP-TON, 1970), the critical function(s) favouring replication of both RV and H-1 virus has to be looked for in the period of cellular DNA synthesis during the cycle. Using parasynchronous cultures of hamster embryo cells RHODE (1973) then showed that, in the case of H-1 virus, initiation of viral DNA synthesis occurred at a specific time in late S-phase only. Moreover, the capacity of rat embryonic cell cultures to support multiplication of RV is affected by low doses of X-ray and UV-irradiation. This is in clear contrast to the sensitivity of other DNA viruses which replicate in the nucleus (TENNANT and HAND, 1970).

(5) *Biochemical Characteristics of Virus Synthesis*

Molecular data concerning the synthesis of viral DNA and proteins are scarcely available*. Using randomly growing rat nephroma cells, SALZMAN and coworkers (1972) found production of RV-DNA to start 8 hours after infection and about 4 hours before infective virions were demonstrable. The latter observation is consistent with results obtained by RHODE (1973, 1974a,b) after parasynchronously multiplying hamster embryo cells had been infected with H-1 virus. In addition, evidence has been presented that in both culture systems continuous synthesis of viral DNA is required for production of viral hemagglutinin. According to sedimentation studies and electron microscopical analysis of nucleic acid molecules extracted from infected cells, replication of the linear single-stranded viral DNA includes a linear double-stranded replicative form (RF). SALZMAN and WHITE suggest this RF-DNA to be formed already within 3 hours after infection, *i.e.* hours before synthesis of progeny DNA molecules starts.

As far as cellular synthetic activity during the period of replication of RV in rat cells is concerned, there is evidence that the rate of protein synthesis remains 75 to 100 per cent and synthesis of RNA is maintained at 100 to 150 per cent of that found in uninfected control cells (SALZMAN et al., 1972). In the same experiments overall DNA synthesis decreased sharply for 6 to 7 hours after infection. Seven to 8 hours p.i., however, DNA synthesis increased again and remained at a high level for the rest of the virus growth period. Finally, multiplication of H-1 and X-14 virus have been reported to alter the level of thymidine kinase—one of the enzymes involved in cellular DNA synthesis—in infected cells (COCUZZA et al., 1967; COCUZZA and COSTARELLI, 1969; FONG et al., 1970). The significance of this effect, however, is still a matter of speculation.

---

* See general survey and addendum.

6. Pathogenesis

a) Natural Hosts

The hamster-osteolytic agents, like most of the other parvoviruses, are viruses in search of a specific disease. Up to the present time, all data concerning their pathogenicity have been obtained only in experimental animal studies, whereas under natural conditions no clear cut relationship between a specific clinical syndrome and any of the isolated viruses could be established. The question of the natural host(s) of the hamster-osteolytic agents, therefore, may be only answered considering the circumstances of isolation and the incidence of specific antibodies found in the assumed host. In this respect, the frequency of direct isolations from rat tissues as well as the high incidence of specific antibodies found in rat populations convincingly suggest the rat as being the natural host for RV and serologically related agents (X-14, H-3, LS, HER, Krisini) as well as for RT-virus. The opinions upon the origin of H-1, HT, and HB-virus, however, are quite controversial. On the basis of her results Toolan concluded these viruses to be of human origin whereas Kilham and Ferm (1964) and Kilham and Margolis (1969) provided evidence for an association of the H-viruses with rats. Above all, these viruses were also considered to be of hamster origin (Nicholson and Hetrick, 1969).

(1) Rat

Besides the history of isolations (cf. section A 1), the high incidence of specific neutralizing and hemagglutination inhibiting antibodies present in rat populations especially suggests this species as being the natural host of RV and serologically related agents. Kilham and Olivier (1959) demonstrated antibodies to RV in the sera of germ-free Lobund rats and Moore and Nicastri (1965), investigating the distribution of the hamster-osteolytic viruses within conventionally raised laboratory rats obtained from various breeders, found evidence for antibodies in a high percentage of sera. Some of the serum samples, in addition, inhibited hemagglutination of H-1 virus. As anti-H-1 activity, however, was always associated with the presence of antibodies to RV, the authors, as Portella (1963) did, supposed this finding to be an effect of hyperimmunization with RV. At present, it is not known whether a similar HI-property directed against H-1 and RV virus may also be found in sera of wild rats, since Robey et al. (1968), examining sera both of laboratory rats (Sprague-Dawley, Fisher, and Wistar strains) and of wild rats (rattus norvegicus and rattus rattus), tested only for anti-RV antibodies. The respective results again pointed to a broad distribution of the agent. Sera of animals from the Wistar- and Fisher-strains as well as those from wild rats proved to be positive in about 50 per cent of the cases while the incidence of specific antibodies in blood samples of Sprague-Dawley rats amounted to 85 per cent.

In an addendum to a more recent paper, Kilham and Margolis (1969) provided strong evidence for the rat being the natural host of H-1 virus, too. On three different occasions the investigators succeeded in isolating a parvovirus with the very characteristics of H-1 virus either from rat embryonic tissue cultures inoculated with rat tissue homogenates or directly from uninoculated control cultures of these cells. Moreover, a high percentage of sera from both wild (76 per

cent) and laboratory rats (80 per cent) was found to contain HI-antibodies to
H-1 virus in relatively high titers of up to 1:320.

(2) Man

The statement of TOOLAN that the H-viruses are of human origin is essentially
based on the frequency of positive isolations after inoculation of human tumors
and other fast growing human tissues into newborn hamsters (TOOLAN et al.,
1962; TOOLAN, 1964; TOOLAN, 1968). The admissibility of this isolation technique
has been repeatedly questioned since a recovery of latent viruses from the inoculated animals cannot be excluded. TOOLAN, however, found this method of
virus detection to be more sensitive than all tissue culture systems tested and,
moreover, showed that numerous blind passages of hamster tumors, embryos, or
tissues in newborn hamsters were negative (TOOLAN, 1961b). Therefore, the ob-
jections made to the thesis of TOOLAN were feeble until KILHAM and MARGOLIS
(1969) reported the successful isolation of H-1 virus from rat tissue cultures after
inoculation of rat tissue homogenates (see section 6, a, 1). Additional negative
evidence also has been presented by NEWMAN and coworkers (1970) who closely
followed the methods of TOOLAN. In contrast to the high frequency of H-virus
isolations from human embryos and placentas (about 20 per cent) recorded by
TOOLAN (1968), these authors failed to isolate any agent out of as many as 50
tissue specimens obtained during spontaneous human abortions. In good accordance with these data, the low incidence of antibodies to H-1 virus so far
found in human sera also would contradict the assumption that man is the
natural host of the H-viruses. Out of 500 serum samples obtained from cancer
patients only „very few" (TOOLAN, 1968) were found to contain antibodies to
H-1 virus and MONIF et al. (1965) who studied sera of 130 women with histories
of spontaneous abortions, stillbirth, and mongolism or congenital defects in their
infants, demonstrated specific antibodies to H-1 in only two serum samples. As
already reported in the previous section, HI-antibodies to H-1, on the contrary,
were present in sera of both wild and laboratory rats at an incidence of about
80 per cent (KILHAM and MARGOLIS, 1969).

b) Experimental Hosts

(1) Rodents

Hamster: Both RV and H-1 virus are of outstanding pathogenicity for newborn hamsters (TOOLAN, 1961a, b; KILHAM, 1961b). Animals infected within
24 hours after birth usually died 4 to 12 days later although only minute doses
of virus had been applied and independent of the route of inoculation. The viruses
can be readily recovered from almost all organs of the infected baby hamsters,
yet, kidneys, liver, and blood yield highest amounts of virus.

With progressive age, however, resistance to the pathogenic action of the
agents increases rapidly. Sucklings inoculated at 4 to 6 days of age frequently
develop only dwarfism and malformations of teeth and bones (cf. section 7b)
rather than a fatally terminating disease. Weanling and adult hamsters finally
are almost insusceptible to infection*. Thus, the observations of KILHAM and
TOOLAN are well in agreement that hamsters after cannibalizing their infected

---

* See addendum.

youngs will only occasionally develop viral antibodies. Experimental inoculation of H-1 virus into adult hamsters, however, was found to result in a cyclic viremia and high titers of infectious virus could be demonstrated in blood samples during the three days following infection as well as on day 9 post inoculation (TOOLAN, 1965). Serum obtained from the animals six days after injection completely neutralized the infectivity of H-1 virus at a dilution of 1 in 320 and detectable amounts of HI-antibodies were present for the first time on day 8 p.i., *i.e.* at the beginning of the second cycle of viremia.

As far as the pathogenicity of the newly isolated RT-virus for hamsters is concerned (SIEGL et al., unpublished), about 10 per cent of the neonates inoculated with virus harvested from tissue cultures died 2—10 days following injection. Successive passages in baby hamsters, however, resulted in an increased and finally stable pathogenicity of RT-virus for the animals. Thus, in passages 4 and 5 all sucklings succumbed on days 4 and 5. Adult animals responded to infection only by formation of antibodies.

Rat: Due to the elevated percentage of animals having antibodies to RV and H-1 virus, rats of all ages frequently resisted experimental infection by the viruses (KILHAM and FERM, 1964). Only after inoculation of high doses of RV into newborn animals specific and occasionally fatal terminating syndromes were seen in a few cases (KILHAM and MOLONEY, 1964; KILHAM and MARGOLIS, 1966; EL DADAH et al., 1967; NOVOTNY and HETRICK, 1970). Even in the proved absence of specific antibodies, the pathogenicity of RV, H-1, and H-3 virus for rats apparently is never a complete one and, moreover, depends largely on the adaptation of the virus to the animals. When MOORE and NICASTRI (1965) injected the agents into specific antibody-free A × C rats, 20 successive passages were necessary before fatal infection of neonates with either virus occurred in more than 50 per cent of the animals 8 days post inoculation.

Mastomy: Besides in hamsters and rats, RV was also found to multiply in the newborn mastomy *(Rattus natalensis)*, an African rodent belonging to the mouse family. Inoculating the virus into neonates of this species, RABSON et al. (1961) tried to induce neoplastic transformation of tissues. Although the experiments in this respect were unsuccessful, the animals developed an acute and lethal disease. Histopathological investigations finally provided evidence that infection of the animals by RV resulted in the formation of intranuclear Feulgen-positive inclusion bodies in cells of the kidneys, liver, spleen, heart, and the lung.

Mouse: KILHAM and OLIVIER (1959) as well as LUM and SCHREINER (1963) noticed that inoculation of RV and the closely related LS-agent into suckling or weanling mice, respectively, never resulted in any clinically apparent disease. Attempts to cultivate the hamster-osteolytic agents in tissue cultures of mouse origin were unsuccessful. For a long time, therefore, the viruses were assumed to be apathogenic for animals of this species. However, EL DADAH et al. (1967) and MATSUO and SPENCER (1969) provided convincing evidence for a quite opposite behaviour.

When EL DADAH et al. (1967) injected concentrated suspensions of HER-agent (at least 10^6 $LD_{50}/0.2$ ml) intracerebrally into 1—2 days old baby mice, they observed development of a fatal paralysis in about 50 per cent of the animals. On the contrary, the sucklings were unaffected after intraperitoneal inoculation with a similar amount of virus. Comparable high virus concentrations also proved to be necessary to demonstrate pathogenicity of RV in BALB/c mice (MATSUO and SPENCER, 1969). Intracerebral inoculation of 10^4 TCID$_{50}$ of RV into baby mice less than 24 hours old resulted either in an acute fatal disease 4 to 8 days post infection or in pronounced dwarfism of the surviving animals. The mortality never amounted to 100 per cent and frequently mice were found devoid of any symptoms at all. There was evidence, however, that the latter animals apparently were latent RV carriers. The agent could be reisolated readily from brain, kidneys, and liver of diseased mice.

(2) Monkey

TOOLAN (1966) could show that both newborn and adult rhesus monkeys *(Macaca mulatta)* are susceptible to infection by H-1 virus. Following subcutaneous inoculation, virus multiplication in adult animals was characterized by viremia and terminated with the formation of neutralizing as well as hemagglutination inhibiting antibodies of relatively low titers (1:80). Only one monkey bearing experimentally induced Rous sarcoma tumors responded with antibody titers as high as 1 in 1280. Similar elevated titers were also recorded when 6 monkeys were injected with H-1 shortly after birth. They all died within three months following inoculation. It proved impossible, however, to attribute death of the animals to virus infection.

Furthermore, TOOLAN (1966) reported that attempts to induce the formation of antibodies to RV, H-3, and HB virus in monkeys were unsuccessful.

(3) Man

That H-1 virus will readily multiply and finally induce formation of specific antibodies in man was demonstrated after injection of the agent into volunteers (TOOLAN et al., 1965). Two female patients—12 and 13 years of age, and suffering from an osteogenic sarcoma whose rapid spread could not be influenced by conventional treatment—were inoculated intramuscularly with H-1 virus. Based on the well known osteolytic effect of the agent in newborn hamsters it was hoped thereby that virus replication would stop further spread of the sarcoma. Daily blood samples were prepared for infectivity tests in newborn hamsters as well as for electron microscopic examination. By means of both methods an apparent cyclic viremia could be demonstrated which was characterized by two virus peaks on days 4 and 9 post inoculation, respectively. Specific neutralizing and hemagglutination inhibiting antibodies were present 10 days after injection. The observed virus multiplication apparently caused the patients no distress; however, it also proved to be without influence on tumor growth.

c) Vertical Transmission of the Viruses

Early in their work concerning the outstanding pathogenicity of H-1 virus for newborn hamsters, TOOLAN and coworkers (1960) noticed that the same type of mongoloid abnormities resulted whether they injected hamster embryos subcutaneously *in utero* 1 to 7 days prior to birth or within 48 hours after birth. A considerable number of the mothers whose fetuses were injected *in utero*, however, aborted or had stillbirths. Stimulated by these observations, TOOLAN et al. inoculated the virus intraperitoneally into 36 pregnant hamsters 1 to 14 days before delivery. Two mothers treated in this way gave birth to a litter, in each of which there was an offspring which later became deformed. The authors, therefore, concluded that H-1 virus was able to cross the placenta and, thus, could induce the well known abnormities *in utero*.

FERM and KILHAM (1964, 1965b) corroborated these findings and described the histopathological changes which accompanied fetal infection with H-1 virus and the spectrum of congenital malformations directly induced by viral action. They found that the severity of the embryocidal and teratogenic effects depended largely on the concentration of the virus-inoculum used. In addition, H-1 virus could be recovered from fetal tissues, and intranuclear inclusion bodies were present in mesodermal tissues such as cartilage, smooth muscle, heart, notochord, meninges of nervous system and especially in the area of the mesodermal somites and mesenchyme of the limb buds. Histological examination also revealed intranuclear inclusions in the trophoblast nuclei of the fetal placentas and in the endodermal cells of the yolk sac placenta.

Intravenous injections of rat virus into pregnant hamsters at different stages of gestation resulted neither in an apparent illness of the mother nor in obvious malformations of the embryos (FERM and KILHAM, 1963; KILHAM and MARGOLIS, 1969). Yet, the agent crossed the placenta and could be recovered from tissues of the uterus, the placenta, and the embryos at significant titers. Fetuses injected *in utero* usually were stillborn or died within hours after parturition.

The first attempts to demonstrate transplacental infection by RV were unsuccessful (KILHAM and FERM, 1964). Shortly afterwards, however, KILHAM and MARGOLIS (1966) reported isolation of a RV strain which, after intraperitoneal inoculation into pregnant Sprague-Dawley rats, led to congenital infection of the fetuses and—depending on the phase of development at which the fetuses were infected—to more or less marked malformations. Inoculation of the mothers late in gestation resulted in cerebellar destruction and severe neonatal hepatitis whilst earlier inoculation produced fetal death or teratogenic effects.

In a study centered at the elucidation of conditions for natural transplacental infection by H-1 and RV in hamsters and rats (KILHAM and MARGOLIS, 1969), one of the main prerequisites for successful infection was found to consist in the use of virus strains which had been subjected to a minimum of laboratory passages only. H-1 viruses then readily passed the placental barrier of pregnant hamsters both after oral and parenteral inoculation as did RV in pregnant rats. Transplacental infection by H-1 in rats, however, could only be achieved by parenteral application of the agent and—vice versa—there was only one special well adapted RV strain found to induce infection of the hamster fetuses by the oral route. The pathways of transplacental infections apparently were different for H-1 and RV. Whereas RV subsequent to inoculation first proliferated in such sites as lung, liver, spleen, as well as in placental tissues of pregnant rats, H-1 virus directly passed the placental barrier in hamsters within 24 hours after oral and parenteral inoculation. In both cases, however, some sort of viremia preceded invasion of the fetuses and the evidently close association of RV and H-1 virus with erythrocytes was supposed to be an effective mechanism for preventing rapid clearance of the virus from the blood stream and, thus, for supporting transplacental infection even in the presence of low amounts of circulating virus.

d) Factors Influencing Pathogenicity

Since TOOLAN presented the first description of the extraordinary alterations induced by H-1 virus after inoculation in neonatal hamsters, many papers dealing with the pathogenicity of RV and H-viruses for small laboratory animals have been published. All reports suggest that in this respect most of the isolates differ in a characteristic manner. As a careful examination of the available data shows, it is, however, not easy to make an objective assessment on the pathogenicity of different strains.

Indeed, extensive studies revealed factors that influence the pathogenic action of the hamster-osteolytic viruses and, hence, caused most of the discrepancies observed. It can be taken for granted that one of these factors is the age, *i.e.* the phase of development at which the animals were infected. Tissues which are actively proliferating during the early neonatal period provide the best conditions for virus multiplication and pathogenicity. As the animal matures the number of tissues which have already acquired their definite structure and function increases and, thus, only restricted tissue areas remain susceptible for the cytopathic action of the virus. Therefore, infection of animals at different phases of development may cause different clinical pictures (cf. section 7).

Furthermore, the history of the virus strain used for injection (*e.g.* number of passages in tissue culture, adaptation to the animal by blind passages) plays an important role. This fact is well illustrated by the findings of KILHAM and FERM (1964) and KILHAM and MARGOLIS (1966, 1969) who noticed that laboratory cultured strains of RV failed to cross the placenta in rats, whereas fresh field strains produced congenital disease after intraperitoneal inoculation. The same investigators (KILHAM and MARGOLIS, 1966) as well as TOOLAN (1968) also observed an increase in virulence of laboratory-grown strains of RV and H-1, respectively, for hamsters during serial passage in animals of this species. Finally, reported variation in pathogenicity may also be due to the dosage of the virus used. This in particular became evident from the results of MATSUO and SPENCER (1969) who attributed their observation that RV—in contrast to previous reports—induced dwarfism and fetal disease in newborn mice, to the inoculation of highly concentrated virus suspensions.

7. Clinical and Pathological Features in Infected Rodents

a) Natural Infection

To our present knowledge, natural infections of rodents by the hamster-osteolytic agents are clinically inapparent and are characterized by the coexistence of persistent virus and antibody. Probably due to the high incidence of antibodies present in populations of both wild and laboratory rats a clear cut relationship between virus infection and a clinically typical syndrome could be never established. From the observations of EL DADAH and coworkers (1967), however, there is strong evidence that a disturbance of the delicate equilibrium existing between the presence of virus and the continued formation of antibodies may convert latent infection into a frank one and, finally, may result in one of the syndromes revealed by experimental studies.

b) Experimental Infection

(1) Acute, Lethal Disease in Newborn Animals

Newborn hamsters proved to be of outstanding susceptibility for infection by the hamster-osteolytic viruses. During successive passages in these animals pathogenicity of H-1 and RV-type viruses could be increased to such an extent that infection as a rule terminated fatally in 50—100 per cent of cases. In baby hamsters infected within 24 hours after birth disease manifested itself 4 to 12 days later by sudden sluggishness and a tendency for the animals to gasp for breath (TOOLAN, 1961b; KILHAM, 1961b). Death usually occurred a few hours after appearance of these symptoms (TOOLAN, 1968). Upon necropsy, hemorrhage of the gut and congestion of the liver were frequent findings.

In case of RT-virus infection of newborn hamsters, the beginning of the disease became apparent as early as 3 days p.i. by occasional appearance of watery feces and, with rapid progress of the illness, was characterized by discharge of blood-stained stools. In about 90 per cent of the dead animals the intestines contained a sanguineous exudate, whereas no characteristic damage of the kidneys, spleen, and liver could be observed (SIEGL et al., unpublished).

When RV, H-3, or H-1 virus were injected into newborn rats, the period of time until death occurred was 7—14 days. Initially the animals showed no symptoms and sucked normally. Only during the last hours before death did they show a certain apathic behaviour and occasionally excretion of bloody feces could be noticed. Autopsy of such rats revealed petechial hemorrhages in the stomach and blood-filled intestines. Histological examination of tissues led to demonstration of intranuclear inclusions in cells of almost all organs of infected animals (MOORE and NICASTRI, 1965).

(2) The Osteolytic Syndrome (Malformation of Teeth and Bones, Dwarfism and Mongolism)

A high percentage of those baby hamsters surviving infection by RV and the H-viruses tended to develop dwarfism frequently associated with mongoloid-like features. To give a suggestive figure, TOOLAN (1960) recorded development of the syndrome in 81 out of 144 survivors. The typical characteristics—small flat face, microcephalic domed head, protruding eyes and tongue, missing or abnormal teeth and fragile bones—could be observed as early as 10—14 days post inoculation. In infected litters of rats and mice the development of dwarfs was rarely found (MOORE, 1963; MOORE and NICASTRI, 1965). With respect to body-weight and size, dwarfish hamsters and rats remained retarded throughout their lives. In mice, however, the differences in size to uninfected controls disappeared with progressive age (MATSUO and SPENCER, 1969).

Already soon after the investigation had been initiated the malformations could be attributed to the exceptional osteolytic activity of the then newly isolated agents. DALLDORF (1060) for the first time described lesions of teeth and bones in hamsters previously inoculated with H-3 virus. Early pathological changes were restricted to the dental pulp and consisted in degeneration of odontoblasts as well as in cystic necrosis of the supporting stroma. Within ten days the teeth became completely destroyed and the dentin developed anomalies.

A thorough study on the relationship between RV infection in hamsters and both growth and condition of the animals' teeth has been presented by BAER and KILHAM (1962a, b; 1964a, b). For this purpose the osteolytic agent was injected intracerebrally into five day old suckling hamsters and the animals were observed for as long as 18 months. By 24 hours post inoculation, edema became evident within the periodontal membrane, the fibroblasts of which could also be shown to contain intranuclear inclusions. Destruction of the periodontal membrane then progressed in such a rapid manner that by day 4 p.i. neither collagenic fibrils nor the supporting alveolar bone was present. Only two to three days later, the space previously occupied by the membrane finally became infiltrated with round cells and, at the same time, resorption of roots as well as bony ankylosis were noted.

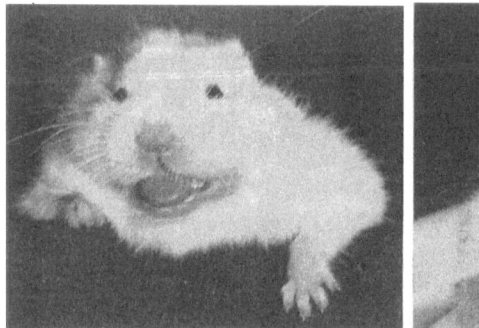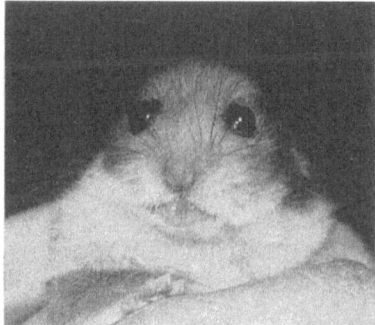

Fig. 1. "Mongoloid-like" hamsters produced by injection of H-1 virus at birth. The animal at the left shows the protruding tongue characteristic for toothless hamsters whereas in the case of the animal at the right the eyes protrude from a microcephalic domed head due to lack of skull space. [From: TOOLAN, HELEN W., Progr. exp. Tumor Res. **16**, 410—425 (1972); courtesy of S. Karger A.G., Basel, Switzerland]

In 16 to 20 day old mongoloid hamsters the pathological changes induced by RV were characterized by advanced resorption of roots and bones, and especially by anomalous depositions of osteodentin and cementum in the region of developing roots of the second molar teeth. Compared with the data in controls, these roots appeared to be shortened and deformed in infected hamsters at 30—60 days of age. A distinct affection of the third molar teeth finally became evident 150 days p.i. and remarkable changes thereby consisted in reduced size of both roots and crowns as well as in necrosis of the pulpa and periapical lesions.

As a result of viral osteolytic activity the denture of 12 to 18 months old hamsters showed some very unusual features. The roots of both the first and second molar teeth had thickened by deposition of a multitude of concentric osteo-cementum layers. Odontogenic "tumors" could be demonstrated within the body of the mandible and about the apical portion of the incisors in the maxilla. Moreover, heavy injury on the growth of alveolar bones, had resulted in exposure of approximately three fourths of the root length of the third molars. The apical third of the root was bulbous and consisted of many concentric layers of osteo-cementum.

According to COHEN and SHKLAR (1964), similar deformities in the denture of the Syrian hamster also occurred after inoculation with H-1 virus. Comparative experiments with RV, H-1, and H-3 virus (BAER and KILHAM, 1965), however, suggested that the three agents could be readily distinguished with respect to frequency and extent of the tooth anomalies induced. It is noteworthy that inoculation of RV led to the least severe malformations.

RV, H-3, and the serologically related Krisini virus as well as H-1 virus in addition were found to affect the development of the skeleton in infected baby hamsters to quite a different extent (FERM and KILHAM, 1965). With H-3 virus, retardation of growth proved to be pronounced in such a way that infected animals gained only 40 per cent of the body weight of uninfected controls. Despite this retardation, however, the proportionality of the skeleton in general remained unaffected, yet, both H-3 and RV showed an obvious affinity for the membranous bones of the skull and the mandible. Due to the presence of lacunae and to missing calcification along cranial sutures, the authors then assumed that the viruses might persist within this region and, thus, are directly responsible for the delay in growth. These findings are well in accordance with the observations of DALLDORF (1960) who, after inoculation of H-3 virus into newborn hamsters, noticed a degeneration of the osteoblasts at the growing costochondral junctions of long bones and attributed the delay in skeletal growth to the same fact.

The osteolytic activity of the aforementioned viruses could not be demonstrated only after inoculation into 1—5 day old baby hamsters. The older the animals had been at the time of infection, however, the fewer malformations became evident. The respective results again suggested the viruses to be of differing osteolytic activity. TOOLAN (1968) frequently noticed malformation of the denture when hamsters were inoculated as weanlings with H-1, H-3, or HT virus but no macroscopic pathogenic affect could be observed when the animals were injected with RV or HB virus. According to histologic studies of BAER and KILHAM (1962b), inoculation of RV into hamsters at 22 days of age resulted in nothing more than resorption and bony ankylosis at the roots of the still developing third molar teeth.

After infection of adult hamsters, the skeleton in general showed no response to the destructive activity of the viruses. Yet, as the investigations of ENGLER et al. (1969) indicated, presence of an osteolytic agent in injured animals may result in a delay in the healing process of osseous wounds. For this purpose the authors injected H-3 virus intravenously into adult hamsters at various intervals following fracture of the forearm or extraction of the maxillary right second molar tooth. Maximum alteration in fracture healing occurred when the virus was injected prior to the third postoperative day and largely consisted in delayed formation of a fibrocartilagenous callus and subperiosteal osteogenesis along the diaphysis. Retardation in osteogenesis was also noticed in alveoli after extraction of teeth when H-3 virus was inoculated into the animals on the first postoperative day. The virus could be readily reisolated from the fracture site. ENGLER et al. therefore suggested the virus either to have a pronounced affinity for those osseous tissues showing an increased mitotic activity or, due to a higher permeability of the blood vessels at the fracture site, to be passively concentrated in this area.

The surprising resemblance between the mongoloid features of deformed hamsters and the human phenotype associated with Down's syndrome as well as the fact that antibodies to H-1 virus could be demonstrated in a mother who gave birth to a mongoloid child (MONIF *et al.*, 1965), caused many speculations on a possible viral etiology of Down's syndrome. Considerations of that kind in addition were stimulated by the statistical inquiries of COLLMAN and STOLLER (1962). For these authors the frequency of Down's syndrome in areas with an elevated density of population and the periodic accumulative appearance of the disease in time intervals of 5—6 years provided suggestive evidence for a viral background. To our present knowledge the syndrome is related to trisomy of the chromosome 21 within the human karyotype. Such an anomaly either may originate from nondisjunction during mitosis or from translocation. GALTON and KILHAM (1966), however, found no indication for a significant chromosome anomaly in cells of deformed hamsters. Moreover, in contrast to the genetic manifestation of the syndrome in man, mongoloid animals gave birth to normal offsprings (TOOLAN, 1960b; FERM and KILHAM, 1965).

(3) *Cerebellar Ataxia*

Within the broad spectrum of clinico-pathological alterations following inoculation of the hamster-osteolytic agents into newborn hamsters and rats there was initially no evidence for involvement of the central nervous system. During pathogenicity testing of four newly isolated strains of RV and of LS agent (LUM and SCHREINER, 1963), KILHAM and MARGOLIS (1964) and MARGOLIS and KILHAM (1966), however, were able to induce cerebellar ataxia in baby hamsters. The typical clinical picture became slowly evident within 4 to 5 weeks subsequent to intracerebral inoculation. In a characteristic manner, the affected animals were smaller than uninfected control animals and developed an unsteadiness of gait as well as an instability of balance. Histopathological examination showed that RV infection selectively attacked the outer germinal layer of the cerebellum and, hence, prevented the formation of the definite cerebellar granular layer. As a result, infection was followed by severe hypoplasia of the cerebellum which subsequently was conserved in the neonatal state.

The syndrome could only be induced when the viruses were inoculated intracerebrally into hamsters less than four days of age, whilst in older animals the cerebellar germinal layers apparently were already insusceptible to infection. The main prerequisite, however, consisted in the use of virus strains little, or not at all, adapted to hamsters. During the first three successive intracerebral passages of two of such virus strains in hamster neonates the agents caused nothing but the described ataxia and intraperitoneal inoculation remained without any effect. Following the third passage, however, virulence of the viruses increased rapidly. Intraperitoneal injection resulted in the development of a hemorrhagic enteritis terminating fatally within 7 to 10 days p.i. After intracerebral inoculation first signs of a severe ataxia developed 12 days post infection. With progressing passage number, the infected animals finally died long before any indication of ataxia could be observed.

Since cerebellar disease following infection of the hamster with RV showed clinical and pathological features similar to spontaneous feline ataxia of kittens

(cf. section E), KILHAM and MARGOLIS (1965) assumed both syndromes to originate presumably from the same etiologic background. Injection of H-1 virus and
various strains of RV, however, revealed that only the RV strain HHP was capable of inducing the anticipated histopathologic alterations in newborn kittens.
Infection with this agent manifested itself as early as 8 days post inoculation by
the appearance of intranuclear inclusions in cells of the cerebellar outer germinal
layer. Simultaneously, a cytopathogenic effect developed resulting in partial destruction of this tissue. Attempts to recover the virus from various tissue specimens of the affected animals also suggested a limitation of virus replication to
the cerebellum. None of the infected kittens, however, developed specific antibodies to RV throughout an observation period of 31 days. According to subsequent studies (KILHAM and MARGOLIS, 1966; JOHNSON et al., 1967) the etiologic
agent of feline ataxia shared many characteristics with the hamster-osteolytic
agents, although these viruses are serologically distinct.

First evidence of cerebellar ataxia in rats was found in a litter of newborn
rats, the mother of which had been inoculated intraperitoneally during pregnancy
with RV strain SpRV (KILHAM and MARGOLIS, 1966). Direct intraperitoneal injection of the agent into newborn animals terminated fatally about 8 days following infection. The cerebellum of the sucklings then frequently showed advanced
lesions and, in one uninoculated baby rat in contact with the infected ones,
typical intranuclear inclusions could be demonstrated in cells of the cerebellar
outer germinal layer.

(4) Hemorrhagic Encephalitis

Special attention should be paid to the pathogenic action of the HER-agent
isolated by EL DADAH et al. (1967) from both brain and spinal cord of adult
Lewis rats after treatment with cyclophosphamide. In contrast to the mere
ataxia syndrome observed after intracerebral inoculation of other strains of RV
into newborn hamsters and rats, this isolate apparently attacked the whole
central nervous system of suckling rats. Affected animals of both species developed specific fatal paralysis and, upon necropsy, severe hemorrhage and necrosis
were noticed in the brain and spinal cord of diseased rats (NATHANSON et al.,
1970; COLE et al., 1970).

8. Immunity

a) Active Immunity

Data concerning the formation of antibodies to the hamster-osteolytic viruses
in the course of a naturally acquired or experimentally induced infection are
only scarcely available. It is well agreed, however, that the onset of experimental
RV or H-1 virus infections in man, hamsters, and rats is characterized by viremia
occurring between 2 to 10 days after inoculation (TOOLAN et al., 1965; TOOLAN,
1965; KILHAM and MARGOLIS, 1969). In general, the end of this viremic phase
coincided with the appearance of detectable amounts of specific humoral antibodies. Thus, in the human, titrable HI-antibodies became evident for the first time
on day 10 whereas serum obtained from hamsters six days after injection completely neutralized the infectivity of H-1 virus at a dilution of 1 in 320. A period
of 7 days finally appears to be the average time necessary for the detection of
HI-antibodies to RV and H-1 virus in rodents.

Once circulating antibodies induced by the hamster-osteolytic agents are present they may persist for a long time at only slowly diminishing or unchanging titers. In the case of a laboratory worker, whose sera were examined over a 4-year period, TOOLAN (1968) observed a constant neutralizing antibody-titer of 1:160 to H-1 virus over a period of three years. The same investigator reported that hamsters injected at birth with H-1 virus and which later became deformed, developed circulating antibodies at titers up to 1:20,000 which remained unchanged throughout the animals' life "of 2—3 years or more" (TOOLAN, 1968). On the other hand, inoculation of the hamster-osteolytic agents into weanling hamsters only resulted in HI-antibody titers of about 1:1280, and to retain this titer level for a longer period, repeated injections of the agents were necessary. A similar behaviour of H-1 antibody titers were noticed after infecting newborn and adult rhesus monkeys (TOOLAN, 1966). With monkeys injected at birth a peak titer of HI-antibodies of 1:2560 was recorded two months after infection. One month later, however, serum obtained from the same animal inhibited hemagglutination of the virus only at a dilution of 1:320. As would be expected, adult rhesus monkeys reacted to a much lesser degree.

In correspondence with the aforementioned data it may be concluded that successful virus multiplication in the tissues of an infected organism (depending on species susceptibility and on completeness of tissue differentiation) is one of the necessities to obtain a reliable antibody response to the injected hamster-osteolytic agent. The repeated isolation of H-1 from livers of mongoloid hamsters with high H-1 antibody titers (TOOLAN, 1960b; 1968) and the recovery of RV from tissues of rats with appreciable levels of RV antibodies (ROBEY et al., 1968), in addition, suggest that the continuous presence of the agents in the animal is a prerequisite for the maintenance of high antibody titers over a long period of time.

The equilibrium existing between latent RV infection in rats and the continuous formation of circulating antibodies obviously is a very delicate one. As EL DADAH and coworkers (1967) showed, a single injection of an immuno-suppressive dose of cyclophosphamide (100 mg/kg) into rats proved to be sufficient to convert a persistent latent RV infection into a clinical apparent disease. Besides this observation, however, the significance of actively acquired immunity after infection with the hamster-osteolytic agents has never been the subject of extensive investigations. KILHAM and FERM (1964) only noticed that circulating antibodies to RV rendered rats of any age relatively insusceptible to inoculation with this agent and RV-"immune" hamsters showed no pathologic response after intracerebral injection of RV-strains which in other cases caused cerebellar ataxia (KILHAM and MARGOLIS, 1964).

TOOLAN (1968), infecting pregnant hamsters and rhesus monkeys with small amounts of H-1 or H-3 virus "certain days before delivery", noticed that none of the mothers produced antibodies to the virus used either after the initial or after repeated injections. She supposed this extraordinary immunological behaviour to be some kind of tolerance occurring in adult animals.

b) Passive Immunity

Considering the pronounced pathogenicity of the hamster-osteolytic agents for fetal tissues and newborn animals, immunity passively transmitted to the embryos *in utero* or to sucklings soon after parturition may be of outstanding significance. In this respect first data were available from a paper of KILHAM and MOLONEY (1964) who showed that suckling rats injected with RV only fell sick when their mothers had no antibodies to the virus. At the same time FERM and KILHAM (1963), injecting RV into pregnant hamsters early in gestation, demonstrated the vertical transmission of the agent and were able to reisolate it from the embryos. With rising titers of maternal antibodies, however, the amount of virus recoverable from fetal tissues decreased. Although it has been well established that in rats maternal antibodies usually are transmitted to the offspring both *in utero* and via colostrum, suckling rats which have been inoculated *in utero* 5—6 days prior to birth, developed—in contrast to the above results—RV infections of equal degree whether or not their mother was free of RV antibodies (KILHAM and FERM, 1964).

9. Epizootiology

The repeated, accidental isolation of RV in many laboratories has already suggested a wide dissemination of the virus in rats and serologic surveys of sera of both laboratory and wild rats strongly support this assumption (MOORE and NICASTRI, 1965; KILHAM, 1966; NATHANSON and COLE, 1968). ROBEY and coworkers (1968) found antibodies to RV in more than 85 per cent of sera collected either from Fisher or Wistar rats. In addition, HI-tests performed with rat sera gathered in Vietnam during a plague study revealed humoral antibody to RV in more than 50 per cent of the species *Rattus norvegicus* and *Rattus rattus*. In the case of H-1 virus, a similar high incidence of specific antibodies could be demonstrated in serum samples obtained from albino rats (KILHAM and MARGOLIS, 1969). This finding is in obvious contrast to the low frequency of antibodies (about 1 per cent) to H-1 and HB-virus in human sera. Considering the fact that presence of antibodies to the hamster-osteolytic agents seems to be always indicative for persistent latent infections, the above data give an impressive picture of the RV and H-1 reservoir constantly available in rat populations.

Corresponding with the latter statement, an observation reported by TOOLAN (1968) looks very meaningful: Germ-free raised weanling Wistar rats, which had no antibodies to either RV or H-1 virus, readily developed antibodies to RV if placed in clean cages in a rat colony room. Since H-1 virus, on the other hand, could be recovered from urine of experimentally infected hamsters, it must be assumed, therefore, that rats bearing a clinically inapparent infection excrete the virus despite the presence of circulating antibodies. The outstanding resistance of the hamster-osteolytic viruses to physical and chemical treatment would then favour their transmission to new hosts via the nasal or the oral route. This mode of virus spread would easily explain the elevated degree of prevalence detected in rat populations. At the present time, however, there is no evidence to answer the question whether all rats "immune" to RV or H-1 virus are permanently excreting infective virus or if there are only some individual excretors. Moreover, the significance of the experimentally proven vertical transmission in the spread of the hamster-osteolytic agents under natural conditions is not known. In any case, RV infections in laboratory animal colonies apparently do not spread via intermediate hosts, since antibodies to the virus were found neither in sera of other animals in contact with rats, *e.g.* mice, guinea pigs, rabbits, and *Suncus muranus* (ROBEY *et al.*, 1968) nor in the sera of workers who cared for the rat colonies (TOOLAN, 1968).

B. The Minute Virus of Mice (MVM)

1. History

The minute virus of mice (MVM) was detected for the first time by CRAWFORD (1966) in stock solutions of mouse adenovirus. This initial observation suggested that MVM might be related to the adeno-associated-satellite viruses but early studies showed the newly isolated agent to be able to replicate in tissue cultures of rat and mouse origin without the presence of a potent helper virus. The isolation of MVM proved to be a stimulus in parvovirus research. CRAWFORD (1966) presented evidence that the nucleic acid of the virus might be a DNA with single-stranded configuration and this, at that time quite uncommon feature of animal viruses, gave rise to the question whether all viruses then classified as "picodnaviruses" would show the same characteristic.

The mere biologic properties and especially the pathogenicity of MVM attracted attention only very recently. It was found that the virus showed as similar a pathogenicity for newborn hamsters as has been reported for the so-called hamster-osteolytic agents (KILHAM and MARGOLIS, '970; PARKER *et al.*, 1970a,b) and, moreover, was highly prevalent in mouse colonies. The observation of KILHAM and MARGOLIS (1970), however, that about 70 per cent of sera collected from both wild and laboratory rats contained HI-antibodies to MVM was questioned by PARKER and coworkers (1970a, b) who attributed the frequent, yet, low antibody titers (1:20—1:40) to the presence of nonspecific inhibitors.

2. Morphology

Electron microscopy of the first density gradient purified preparation of MVM revealed closely packed arrays of uniform particles with approximately hexagonal outlines. After negative staining, maximum and minimum center to center distances between particles in this aggregate of 26 and 19 nm were measured suggesting a particle size fitting well to that of the other parvoviruses. During subsequent studies, CRAWFORD's group reported a diameter of 28 ± 1 nm, and comparative examination of adeno-associated virus type 1 (AAV-1) led to the same size.

The ultrastructure of MVM has not yet been resolved. Occasionally electron micrographs showed particles having an electron-dense core which obviously resulted from penetration of the negative stain into the virus particle. Data on the diameter of this core, however, are not available.

3. Physicochemical Characteristics

a) Configuration of Nucleic Acid

The DNA nature of MVM nucleic acid has been well established by tracer analysis (CRAWFORD *et al.*, 1969). First evidence for a single-stranded configuration of the molecule could be obtained by CRAWFORD (1966) when the reaction of formaldehyde with purified MVM preparations in analogy to the observations with phage ΦX-174 (SINSHEIMER, 1959) and denatured double-stranded DNA resulted in a shift of the UV-absorption maximum of the virus towards a longer wavelength. It had to be concluded, therefore, that the amino groups of the bases in MVM-DNA are not occupied by hydrogen bonding between base pairs. Moreover, buoyant density centrifugation of extracted MVM-DNA in the presence of double-stranded bacterial DNA of known properties at both pH 8.5 and 12.5 — where the DNA's would have undergone strand separation — indicated single-stranded configuration. The constantly observed density of 1.722 g/ml corresponded to a content of guanine plus cytosine (GC) of about 48 per cent. As it was found with ΦX-174 phage DNA (SCHILDKRAUT et al., 1962), the actual value of GC determined by tracer experiments proved to be lower (41 per cent) than that predicted from buoyancy. In respect to the high thymine content of the DNA, the latter results also revealed a striking similarity between MVM-DNA and the single-stranded DNA's of the phages ΦX-174, fd, and M 13. In addition, the reported base composition (CRAWFORD et al., 1969) pointed to single-stranded configuration since in MVM-DNA a significant condition of double-stranding — adenine should equal thymine and guanine should equal cytosine — is not satisfied*.

Electron miscroscopy of extracted MVM-DNA prepared by the Kleinschmidt-technique (KLEINSCHMIDT and ZAHN, 1959) revealed molecules having a mean length of 1.2 μ. On the basis of a mass per unit length of 1.25×10^6 daltons/μ derived from the size of ΦX-174 DNA as determined in parallel experiments and from its known molecular weight (1.7×10^6; SINSHEIMER, 1959a), the molecular weight of MVM-DNA finally was calculated to be 1.5×10^6 daltons.

b) Buoyant Density and Sedimentation Behaviour

For the complete, fully infectious virion of MVM buoyant density values in CsCl varying between 1.41 and 1.43 g/ml were recorded. These figures are compatible with average densities determined for other parvoviruses such as RV for which a density range of 1.37—1.47 g/ml can be deduced from the data reported. With other parvoviruses, isopycnic centrifugation studies usually revealed an additional zone of low infectivity but high hemagglutinating activity at densities of 1.30—1.32 g/ml besides the band containing fully infective virus. A band with similar properties has also been observed after isopycnic banding of MVM. In contrast to the latter data, however, its mean density was determined to be 1.35 g/ml. Since this value is much higher than the one expected for a simple protein, CRAWFORD suggested the "empty" virus particles detected by electron microscopic examination of these gradient fractions to contain at least some residual nucleic acid. The occasional resolution of a further band at an intermediate density of 1.38 g/ml strongly supports this assumption.

MVM sediments at the same rate of 110 ± 2 S as RV and H-1 virus (McGEOCH et al., 1970).

---

* See addendum.

4. Antigenic Structure and Serologic Properties

There is no indication that the antigenic structure of MVM may be distinct from that of other parvoviruses capable of independent replication. Both hemagglutinating and complement-fixing properties of the virus have been detected and, from correlated investigation of gradient fractions by hemagglutination and electron microscopy, it also may be concluded that the hemagglutinating ability is bound to the protein subunits of the particle's capsid.

According to CRAWFORD (1966), MVM hemagglutinin has a pronounced affinity for red blood cells of guinea pig, hamster, rat, and mouse origin at temperatures between 4° and 37° C, whereas with sheep, fowl, and human red blood cells under similar conditions extremely low hemagglutinating titers could be recorded. These results are largely consistent with the MVM-hemagglutination spectrum observed by HALLAUER et al. (1972) who noticed quite good agglutination of human, guinea pig, mouse, rat, hamster, and dog erythrocytes. Insignificant or negative results, however, were obtained with red blood cells of rhesus monkey, rabbit, sheep, horse, cattle, pig, cat, fowl, and goose origin (cf. Table 8, p. 88).

According to the results of cross hemagglutination-, neutralization-, and complement-fixation tests, MVM is serologically unrelated to H-1, H-3, RV, PPV, and HALLAUER's virus strains (CRAWFORD, 1966; KILHAM and MARGOLIS, 1970; HALLAUER et al., 1971; CROSS and PARKER, 1972) (cf. Table 9, p. 90). Immunofluorescent studies, however, suggested some antigenic relationship with H-1 and RV: MVM infected rat embryonic cells were stained by both H-1 and RV antibody, but MVM antibody did not bind to cells containing RV or H-1 (CROSS and PARKER, 1972).

5. Growth Characteristics

a) Cultivation

MVM was shown to grow in primary mouse lung and in primary or secondary monolayer cultures of rat and mouse embryo cells (CRAWFORD, 1966; PARKER et al., 1970). Although observed in both rat and mouse cells, CPE was more prevalent in cultures of rat origin. The cytologic changes were indistinguishable from those described for the hamster-osteolytic viruses. HALLAUER and coworkers (1972) succeeded in growing MVM in permanent cell lines of rat (AT), mouse (L), and hamster (BHK-21 and BHK-35) origin. Multiplication of the virus in these culture systems was accompanied by vague, but nevertheless specific cytopathic changes mostly consisting of rounding up of cells and detaching of the cell sheet. Attempts to cultivate MVM in permanent strains of human, monkey, pig, and rabbit cells failed.

Recently, a plaque assay for MVM in A-9 cell cultures (a cell strain derived from the mouse L cell line) was developed by TATTERSALL (1972b). Previous experiments had provided evidence that propagation of the virus in actively growing cells led to about 10 times as much infectious units as could be recovered after infection of a resting cell sheet. Therefore, the cultures were infected at the time of cell seeding. The developing plaques were of variable diameter ranging between 1 and 8 mm. It could be shown that this variation in plaque size was not a genetically controlled one but depended largely on the initial cell density used in the test.

b) Virus Multiplication

According to observations following immunofluorescent staining, both the cytoplasm and the nucleus of infected cells are involved in MVM replication (PAR-KER et al., 1970a). The experimental conditions applied did not allow a clear cut correlation between the recognized localization of stainable antigen and the time course of the virus synthesis; yet, the majority of intracytoplasmic antigen appeared concomitant with the decrease of intranuclear fluorescence. The predominance of the nucleus in virus replication is finally supported by the observation that staining of infected monolayers with May-Grünwald-Giemsa revealed intranuclear inclusions.

Comparable to the findings with RV and H-1 virus, progress of MVM multiplication depends on host cell function(s) and, very likely, is controlled by synthetic events occurring in late S-phase of the cell cycle (TATTERSALL, 1972b). Under optimum conditions, viral replication was suggested to extent for 12 to 15 hours (DOBSON and HELLEINER, 1973). The rate of cellular DNA synthesis—measured in cultures of randomly growing cells—proved to be only slightly altered following infection with MVM. About 14 hours p.i., however, a "considerable proportion" of intracellular DNA was found to consist of a double-stranded replicative form and of single-stranded progeny viral DNA (TATTERSALL, 1972a, b; DOBSON and HELLEINER, 1973)*.

6. Pathogenesis

a) Natural Host(s)

In close similarity to the characteristics of natural RV-infections in rats, MVM-infections in colonies of the accepted natural host, the mouse, apparently are highly prevalent, however, persist only in a clinically inapparent state. PARKER and coworkers (1970b) tested sera of mice from 52 conventional and SPF breeder colonies 79 per cent of which contained HI-antibodies to the virus with titers occasionally exceeding 1:1000. Moreover, 76 (20 per cent) of 390 sera collected from wild mice (Mus musculus) in four different states of the United States showed HI-titers in the range from 1:20 to 1:160. From 8 mice having HI-antibody titers higher than 1 in 100 and being 40—45 days of age, MVM could be recovered from the kidneys or from blood in 7 and 3 cases, respectively. This result strongly suggests a coexistence of infective MVM and specific antibody in mice in good agreement with the observations reported for other parvoviruses.

After experimental inoculation into newborn mice, MVM proved to be pantropic, yet, proliferated to highest titers in brains (KILHAM and MARGOLIS, 1970). None of the infections terminated fatally and the only clinically apparent effect consisted in growth retardation of inoculated animals compared with uninoculated littermate controls. The cerebellum of all examined mice showed "mild or moderate" lesions in the external germinal layer. Clinical ataxia, however, was never observed.

PARKER and coworkers (1970b) tested a total of 2874 sera from other rodents including rats (1550), hamsters (747), rabbits (346), guinea pigs (76), gerbils (50),

---

* See general survey.

and lemmings (105) for HI-antibodies to MVM. Positive results were only obtained with sera of rats. Although the overall incidence of HI-potency in these samples was very high, individual titers usually did not exceed 1:40, and could be reduced by treatment with receptor destroying enzyme. In contrast to KILHAM and MARGOLIS (1970) who had obtained comparable positive results with 69.5 per cent of sera of wild rats, PARKER *et al.* therefore questioned whether the observed hemagglutination-inhibition really was due to MVM-antibodies. Moreover, attempts to recover the virus from 114 rats having positive HI-titers failed.

b) Experimental Hosts

Rat: In contrast to the unresolved question concerning the role of rats in natural MVM-infections, there is no doubt that experimental (i.p. and i.c.) inoculation of the virus into neonates of this species results in a reproductive, yet, subclinical infection (KILHAM and MARGOLIS, 1970). Reliable amounts of virus could be recovered on day 7 post injection from brain, liver, gut, blood, and urine of the sucklings. Pathologic effects were restricted to the ependyma and choroid plexus both showing mild cytolytic effects and presence of intranuclear inclusions.

Hamster: Newborn hamsters injected within 48 hours after birth show the most severe clinical reactions to infection by MVM (KILHAM and MARGOLIS, 1970). Onset of disease was usually indicated by the presence of an anal exudate between 5 and 8 days following inoculation and, in heavily affected animals, disease frequently terminated fatally on day 6. MVM could be reisolated at relative high titers from a pool of livers, spleens, kidneys, and brains of dead animals.

Hamsters surviving MVM infection were retarded in growth in comparison with uninoculated controls and occasionally had features of mongolism and peridontal disease comparable to those described for the hamster-osteolytic viruses (cf. chapter A).

c) Transmission

As evident from the above sections, MVM could be readily recovered from both blood and gut of experimentally infected mice and rats, and, moreover, was found to be excreted in urine. On the basis of these observations, dissemination of MVM within colonies of these species by the fecal-oral route appears to be the most probable one. By means of experiments designed to elucidate the significance of several routes of virus transmission in mouse colonies, PARKER and coworkers (1970b) found that mice in close contact with infected donor animals developed antibodies to MVM at the same rate as did those contaminated only by urine and feces. After limited contact (nasal-oral) the antibody response of uninoculated test mice proved to be retarded and after separating the cages of infected and uninfected animals by an 8 inch airspace no reaction at all could be observed.

According to KILHAM and MARGOLIS (1971), MVM may also spread in mice by transplacental transmission. In addition, MOHANTY and BACHMANN (1974) were able to infect fertilized two-celled mouse eggs. However, virus multiplication had no deliterious effect on development of embryos cultivated *in vitro*.

C. Porcine Parvovirus (PPV)

1. History

Dealing with the multiplication of hog cholera virus in primary and secondary tissue cultures of pig origin, MAYR and MAHNEL (1964, 1966) found themselves faced with the problem of latent viruses present in these cells. Many of the pig kidney cultures (PK-cultures) used contained porcine adenovirus (MAHNEL and BIBRACK, 1966) and electron microscopic examination of culture media collected from both hog cholera-infected PK- and piglet testicle cell cultures also revealed a 22—23 nm sized particle, the morphology of which MAHNEL (1965) reported to be "very similar to those of foot-and-mouth-disease virus and Kilham rat virus". These findings were corroborated by HORZINEK et al. (1967) who also stated that the small particle may contain deoxyribonucleic acid. Finally, MAYR and co-workers (1968) were able to isolate the virus from several batches of uninoculated primary monolayer cultures of kidneys from healthy three week old pigs and found it to share many characteristics with members of the parvovirus group.

Further evidence for the occurrence of a small porcine DNA-virus has been provided during studies concerning the viral etiology of herd infertility, abortions, and stillbirths in pigs (CARTWRIGHT and HUCK, 1967). Thereby, of 111 attempts 96 proved to be successful in isolating a small sized, ether resistant, and DNA containing virus. Serological investigations (CARTWRIGHT et al., 1969) suggested that this virus is identical with, or at least closely related to, the agents isolated by MAYR and coworkers (1968), DARBYSHIRE and ROBERTS (1968) as well as to "Wavre"-virus, previously supposed by HUYGELEN and PEETERMANS (1967) to be a hemagglutinating ECSO-virus. Despite the frequency of isolations and the extensive attempts to demonstrate some correlation between presence of PPV and cases of reproductive failure (e.g. JOHNSON, 1969a and b), the etiological role of the virus is still in question. Nevertheless, serological surveys of serum samples gathered in Canada, the United Staates, Holland, Northern Ireland, Germany, and Switzerland, strongly support the assumption that PPV infections presumably are common in normally raised pig stock all over the world.

2. Morphology

The morphological characteristics of PPV resemble those described for the hamster-osteolytic agents. From electron micrographs its diameter was estimated to be 20 to 28 nm (HORZINEK et al., 1967; MAYR et al., 1968; CARTWRIGHT et al., 1969) and the same size could be calculated from ultrafiltration experiments. The exact structure of PPV has not been investigated. Capsomeres were demonstrated only occasionally. In negative stained, closely packed aggregates of PPV, however, HORZINEK et al. (1967) and MAYR et al. (1968) observed particles with hexagonal outline. From this, the latter investigators concluded that the virus may be of icosahedral symmetry. On the other hand, HORZINEK et al. felt that the narrow zone of dispersion recorded during statistical evaluation of the agent's diameter points to central symmetric configuration. Electron microscopy of ultrathin sections of PPV infected pig kidney cells only revealed the well stained nucleoprotein containing core of the virus (MAYR et al., 1968). As it has been observed with RV and H-1 virus, this core measured about 15 nm in diameter (SIEGL, 1969, unpublished observation).

3. Physicochemical Characteristics

a) Type of Nucleic Acid

The DNA nature of the nucleic acid present in the core of PPV has only been established on the basis of results obtained by use of DNA antagonists and acridine orange staining. CARTWRIGHT and HUCK (1967), as well as MAYR et al. (1968), reported significant inhibition of virus multiplication in pig kidney monolayers after the addition of either 5-iodo-deoxyuridine or 5-bromodeoxy-uridine to the culture media. Since control experiments—including pseudorabies virus (DNA) and Teschen disease virus (RNA)—clearly confirmed the selective inhibitory action of the compounds for DNA viruses, the authors suggested PPV to contain DNA. Attempts to estimate the nucleic acid type by means of acridine orange staining of concentrated virus suspensions according to the method of MAYOR and DIWAN (1961) were rather inconclusive. HORZINEK et al. (1967) were only able to state that pretreatment with pepsin and DNase prevented staining of the virus. There was, however, no indication whether PPV contains single- or double-stranded DNA.

Many of the virus strains isolated by HALLAUER and coworkers (1971) from permanent human cell lines proved serologically indistinguishable from the PPV strain originally described by MAYR et al. (1968) (see chapter G and Table 9). The DNA of KBSH-virus, a reference strain of these contaminants, has been characterized by SIEGL (1972) and, very likely, the values obtained may be relevant for PPV. According to these results, PPV contains a linear, single-stranded DNA with a molecular weight of 1.4×10^6 daltons and a GC content of 48 per cent. Both native and denatured DNA of KBSH-virus was described to sediment around 24S in neutral solution. It could be recovered from CsCl gradient fractions having a density of 1.724 g/ml. Finally, the molecular weight of the DNA was calculated to amount to 26.5 per cent of a total virus particle weight of 5.3×10^6 daltons.

b) Buoyant Density

In density gradient studies with tissue culture material containing hog cholera virus and porcine adenovirus in addition to PPV, the three agents could be easily separated by isopycnic banding in CsCl. Whereas adenovirus and hog cholera virus banded in a density range of 1.32—1.34 and 1.15—1.20 g/ml, respectively (MAHNEL et al., 1967; HORZINEK and UEBERSCHAER, 1966; MAYR et al., 1967), peak titers of infective PPV were found in fractions having a medium density of 1.37—1.39 g/ml (HORZINEK et al., 1967; MAYR et al., 1968). Testing the gradient for distribution of hemagglutinating activity of PPV revealed a further peak present at a density of about 1.32—1.33 g/ml (HORZINEK et al., 1968). However, infectivity of these fractions was very low (MAYR et al., 1968).

c) Resistance to Physical and Chemical Agents

(1) Heat

Incubation of cultured PPV at 56° C for 30 minutes resulted neither in a reduction of infectivity nor in a significant change of the hemagglutinating ability of the virus (CARTWRIGHT and HUCK, 1967; MAYR et al., 1968). Samples still proved to be infective even after incubation at 70° C for 2 hours but infectivity apparently was lost at 80° C after 5 minutes (CARTWRIGHT et al., 1969). At temperatures higher than 75° C the hemagglutination titers recorded also declined to almost zero (SIEGL et al., 1969, unpublished).

(2) pH-Stability

CARTWRIGHT and HUCK (1967) noticed that strain 59 E/63 of PPV appeared to be acid-resistant and MAYR et al. (1968) reported stability of the agent in a range of pH 3 − 9. Infectivity disappeared completely at pH 2 after incubation at 37° C for 90 minutes. In agreement with the latter observation, SIEGL and coworkers (1969, unpublished) found that hemagglutination titers of PPV suspensions at extreme pH values, i.e. pH-2 and pH-9 declined after 30 minutes incubation at temperatures above 37° C.

(3) Organic Solvents

The virus proved to be insensitive to treatment with ether and chloroform (CARTWRIGHT and HUCK, 1967; MAYR et al., 1968). In addition, concentration of PPV from tissue culture harvests by use of methanol precipitation and chloroform/butanol extraction gave good results (MAHNEL, 1965).

(4) Trypsin

Treatment of PPV with trypsin for 1 hour did not reduce the infectivity titers of virus suspensions. On the contrary, a small but regular rise of the titers occurred which, perhaps, can be attributed to the dispersion of virus aggregates (MAYR et al., 1968).

(5) Storage at Low Temperature

PPV stored in tissue culture medium or glycine buffer (pH 9.0) at − 20° and − 70° C for 6 and more than 12 months showed no loss in infectivity and hemagglutinin titer (CARTWRIGHT et al., 1969; SIEGL, unpublished observation).

4. Antigenic Structure

PPV suspensions derived from infected monolayer cultures were shown to contain neutralizable, hemagglutinating, and complement-fixing antigens (HORZINEK et al., 1967; CARTWRIGHT and HUCK, 1967; MAYR et al., 1968; HALLAUER et al., 1972). The hemagglutinating antigen is recovered from gradient fractions containing either infectious or noninfectious, sometimes disrupted virus particles. Data concerning the nature of the complement-fixing antigen are not available.

The range of agglutinated red blood cells from various animal species is listed in Table 8 (p. 88). In general, a rather broad spectrum of well agglutinable erythrocytes of rodent, higher mammalian, and avian origin has been found.

Less susceptible RBC's — e.g. those of sheep, dog, cat, mouse, and goose — are still agglutinated but higher concentrations of PPV were necessary to obtain the same effect. Hemagglutination readily occurred at room temperature; according to MAYR et al. (1968), however, most consistent results could be obtained after incubating the test tubes for 5—6 hours at +4° C.

Serologically, PPV is closely related to KBSH-virus which has been isolated from permanent human cell lines by HALLAUER et al. (1971) but shares no antigen in common with other parvoviruses (cf. Table 9, p. 90).

5. Cultivation

a) Host-Cell Range

PPV was shown to multiply and to induce specific cytopathic effects in cell cultures of pig origin (CARTWRIGHT and HUCK, 1967; MAYR et al., 1968; CARTWRIGHT et al., 1969). Primary and subcultured cell monolayers were found as suitable as stable porcine kidney cell lines. Since, however, according to serologic investigations (cf. section 6) latent PPV infections are wide spread in pig stocks, stable cell lines known to be free of contaminating viruses should be preferred.

Calf kidney and calf testicle cells proved to be insusceptible to PPV and MAYR and coworkers (1968) did not succeed in cultivating the virus in established cell lines of human, monkey, and rat origin. In contrast to this observation, CARTWRIGHT et al. (1969) and HALLAUER et al. (1972) noticed that the human cell lines HEp-2, HeLa, Lu 106, Lu 132, and KB supported growth of the virus and, as far as HeLa and KB cells are considered, multiplication of the virus was accompanied by a vague but specific cytopathic effect.

b) Cytopathogenicity and Virus Multiplication

Both multiplication of PPV and the appearance of specific cytopathic alterations are favoured by the presence of large numbers of dividing cells in infected cultures. Thus, MAYR et al. (1968) and CARTWRIGHT and coworkers (1969) obtained best results when the virus was added to porcine kidney monolayers "not yet completely confluent". HALLAUER et al. (1972) observed the highest rate of virus replication when inoculating PPV simultaneously with or only a short time after seeding of the cells.

Cytopathic effect was usually characterized by diffuse granulation, rounding up of cells and, finally, partial or complete detachment of the destroyed cell sheet from the glass surface. When rapidly growing cultures were infected at a relative high multiplicity, the first signs of CPE could be noticed 2—5 days post inoculation. Monolayers infected with small amounts of virus developed similar cytopathic changes only after repeated subculturing the infected cells (CARTWRIGHT et al., 1969; HALLAUER et al., 1972). In addition, HALLAUER and coworkers demonstrated that PPV specific hemagglutinin could be recovered—by the alkaline extraction technique—from HeLa and KB cultures inoculated with highly diluted virus samples and not showing CPE after more than 10 days. The determination of endpoint dilutions by means of extraction of hemagglutinin therefore yielded higher titers than did the reading of cytopathic changes.

Staining of infected pig kidney cultures with hematoxylin/eosin revealed type A intranuclear inclusion bodies as early as 18 to 24 hours post inoculation. The inclusions usually filled the whole nucleus leaving only space for the marginated nucleoli (CARTWRIGHT and HUCK, 1967; MAYR et al., 1968). Immunofluorescent studies suggested the intranuclear inclusion to consist of viral antigen (DANNER and BACHMANN, 1968, personal communication; CARTWRIGHT et al., 1969; LUCAS and NAPHTINE, 1971) and, according to microscopic examination of ultrathin sections, the infected nuclei contain closely packed arrays of virus particles in the interchromatine area (MAYR et al., 1968).

The appearance of intranuclear inclusion bodies as early as 18 hours following infection and the linear accumulation of both hemagglutinating and infective virus between 8 and 24 hours p.i. finally suggest the replication cycle of PPV in actively growing cells to extent for about 18 to 24 hours (BACHMANN, 1972).

6. Pathogenicity

Observations reported on the pathogenicity of the virus are mostly restricted to only one animal of interest, the pig. The few experimental studies dealing with the susceptibility of further hosts (MAYR et al., 1968; CARTWRIGHT et al., 1969) such as embryonated hen's eggs, newborn as well as suckling hamsters and mice were negative. Because of the small number of animals tested and lacking successive blind passages, however, this failure may be not definite.

In contrast to this, the role of the pig as the natural host for PPV has been very well established. CARTWRIGHT and HUCK (1967) surveyed the sera of 430 pigs, collected from abattoirs and farms in England and Scotland, for hemagglutination-inhibiting antibody to PPV and found 33 per cent to have positive titers. Similar results were obtained in Germany (BACHMANN, 1969) and the United States (MENGELING, 1972). JOHNSON and COLLINGS (1969) even reported 50 to 90 per cent of pigs from different stocks in England as having both HI- and neutralizing antibodies to PPV. Moreover, the wide spread occurrence of PPV in pigs is supported by the frequent recovery of the virus directly from cell cultures of pig origin as well as from cell cultures inoculated with homogenates of pig tissue specimens (CARTWRIGHT and ROBERTS, 1968; MAYR et al., 1968; BACHMANN, 1969; JOHNSON, 1969a; CARTWRIGHT et al., 1969).

All these observations are mainly concerned with clinically latent infections, whereas the significance of PPV infections in porcine disease is still a matter of speculation. CARTWRIGHT and HUCK (1967), interested in the viral etiology of herd infertility, abortions, and stillbirth in pigs, recovered PPV from 96 out of 111 samples of tissues, vaginal mucus, and semen from infected herds and, hence, supposed the virus to play an important role in pig reproductive failure. In addition, PPV was found associated with pneumonitis and could be isolated from nasal turbinates during a study of naturally occurring rhinitis of swine (DARBYSHIRE and ROBERTS, 1968; MENGELING, 1972). Further studies showed, however, that the virus as readily may be recovered from tissues of normal healthy pigs as from stillborn and aborted piglets or from animals suffering from respiratory disease (JOHNSON, 1969; JOHNSON and COLLINGS, 1969, 1971; CARTWRIGHT et al., 1969, 1971).

Experimental studies led to only little more additional information*. They revealed that infection of both antibody-free piglets and pregnant gilts by different routes (oral, intranasal, intramuscular, intravenous) was followed by viremia and low grade leukopenia from days one through five post inoculation

---

* See addendum.

(JOHNSON and COLLINGS, 1969). Specific HI- and neutralizing antibodies to PPV could be detected for the first time 6 to 9 days after injection but none of the animals developed any specific clinical signs of illness (MAYR et al., 1968; JOHNSON and COLLINGS, 1969; BACHMANN, 1969; CARTWRIGHT et al., 1971). No reliable indication for embryocidal or teratogenic effects of PPV could be recorded*. Successful reisolation from tissues of apparently normal offspring and from occasional stillborn piglets, however, clearly demonstrated vertical transmission of the virus.

7. Immunity

After inoculation of PPV into antibody-free pigs, significant HI- and neutralizing antibody titers could be demonstrated as early as 6 to 9 days post inoculation, and 14 to 21 days p.i., titers of 1024—5000 were recorded (MAYR et al., 1968; BACHMANN, 1969; JOHNSON and COLLINGS, 1969; CARTWRIGHT et al., 1971). Similar HI-titers were found in sera of uninfected littermate pigs kept in close contact with infected animals.

BACHMANN (1969a, b) reported distribution pattern of HI-antibodies in pigs of different ages. The most striking result thereby consisted in the high incidence (92.5 per cent) of rather elevated antibody titers (1:744) in suckling piglets. The significantly reduced HI-titers (1:134) and the decreased percentage of positive sera (78.3 per cent) recorded for pigs of 4 to 6 weeks advanced age strongly suggested these original high antibody levels to reflect a status of passive immunity. On the other hand, JOHNSON and COLLINGS (1969) as well as CARTWRIGHT et al. (1971), who infected dams in pregnancy or inoculated embryos in utero, noticed elevated levels of both HI- and neutralizing antibodies in newborn piglets before suckling. The antibody titers remained high in these animals whether the piglets were reared with or without colostrum. Since it is known that newborn pigs very early in their lives are capable of antibody formation (KIM et al., 1964) and considering the fact that in pigs passive immunity is only transmitted via colostrum, the aforementioned observations may be only ascribed to actively acquired immunity.

In close resemblance to conditions recorded for other parvoviruses, actively acquired immunity to PPV in adult pigs apparently also persists due to a coexistence of latent virus infection and demonstrable antibody. The results of BACHMANN (1969) who, in five cases, was able to isolate the virus from kidneys of pigs, all of which had specific HI-antibodies up to titers of 1:2048, points at least in this direction.

D. Feline Panleukopenia Virus (FPV)

(Syn.: Feline enteritis, Feline agranulocytosis virus, Feline ataxia virus, Mink enteritis virus.)

1. History

When in 1966 JOHNSON and CRUICKSHANK presented first evidence that the causative agent of feline panleukopenia might presumably be a member of the newly established parvovirus-group, they were beginning to write the last chapter

---

* See addendum.

of the story about a fatal feline disease in which bacteriologists, pathologists, as well as virologists have been interested since the end of the 19th century. Moreover, the following studies of JOHNSON and his coworkers gave rise to the assumption that such fairly distinct clinical pictures as feline enteritis, mink enteritis, feline panleukopenia, and feline ataxia are due to only one and the same infectious agent.

The intensive investigations aimed at the isolation of the causative agent of infectious feline enteritis were started in 1900 by ZSCHOKKE who at frequent occasions recovered *E. coli* from affected cats. The bacteriologic etiology had to be put aside, however, when VERGE and CHRISTOFERONI (1928) showed that the disease could be induced and passaged in healthy animals by organ emulsions filtered through bacteria-tight Berkefeld candles. Subsequent filtration experiments of HINDLE and FINDLAY (1932) as well as of URBAIN (1933) finally confirmed the suggestion that the syndrome might be caused by a virus.

Between 1938 and 1943 experimental research was centered especially on the clinico-pathologic features of feline infectious enteritis. The studies then revealed that, besides an almost constant involvement of the intestine, the main characteristic regularly consisted in a severe alteration of the blood picture. Based on the hematological changes they believed to be the most characteristic ones, the various investigators proposed a specific name for the syndrome. LAWRENCE and SYVERTON (1938, 1940) referred to "feline agranulocytosis", HAMMON and ENDERS (1939 a, b) to "feline panleukopenia", and KIKUTH and coworkers (1940) to "infectious aleukocytosis". By means of comparative pathological examinations as well as by cross protection tests, however, LAWRENCE *et al.* (1943) and LUCAS and RISER (1945) were able to show that all the different syndromes and perhaps some cases of the really obscure disease "feline distemper" are caused by the same virus.

During the studies reported above, attempts to infect animals other than members of the family *Felidae* had failed (URBAN, 1933; HAMMON and ENDERS, 1939; KIKUTH *et al.*, 1940). It therefore attracted considerable interest, when in Canada during 1947 and 1950—1952 serious epizootics of enteritis with clinical features similar to infectious feline enteritis occurred among ranch mink (SCHOFIELD, 1949; WILLS, 1952). The virus nature of the etiologic agent could be again ascertained by filtration experiments. Moreover, it proved possible to induce the syndrome in mink by experimental infection with feline panleukopenia virus (FPV) (MACPHERSON, 1956; MYERS *et al.*, 1959 b), and WILLS and BELCHER (1956), as well as MYERS *et al.* (1959 b), and BURGER *et al.* (1963, 1964) succeeded in demonstrating a close serologic relationship between FPV and mink enteritis virus (MEV) by means of cross protection tests.

In the past ten years, the successful propagation of FPV and MEV in tissue cultures of feline origin (GORHAM *et al.*, 1965, 1966; JOHNSON 1964, 1965, 1966, 1967) finally provided a reliable basis for a thorough investigation of the viruses' properties. Convincing results revealed a close resemblance of the *in vitro* behaviour of both agents and, in addition, proved definitely their serologic identity (JOHNSON, 1967; JOHNSON *et al.*, 1967). Above all, the morphology as well as the physicochemical characteristics of FPV/MEV justifying a membership of the virus in the parvovirus group could now be readily determined (JOHNSON *et al.*, 1974).

The last significant event in the history concerning FPV/MEV consisted in the discovery that this virus also causes the ataxic syndrome of newborn kittens which for a long time was believed to be of genetic origin (KILHAM and MARGOLIS, 1966; JOHNSON et al., 1967).

2. Morphology

JOHNSON and CRUICKSHANK (1966) succeeded in determining the approximate size of FPV and MEV by successive filtration of tissue-cultured viruses through filters of 80, 45, and 39 nm average pore size. Thereby, culture harvests ultra-sonicated only once before filtration usually failed to pass an 80 nm APD membrane. After repeated ultrasonic treatment, however, the infective agent readily passed a 45 nm filter but was held back by a 39 nm one, thus suggesting a particle size of 27—35 nm. Confirmation of virus size and a presumable explanation for the unusual filtration behaviour of the agent finally has been provided by electron microscopic examination of the virus suspension. With few exceptions, only aggregates composed of small particles about 20 nm in diameter were found in negative stained preparations. It then seemed logical that only after ultrasonic disruption of the clumps, single infective particles could pass the 80 and 45 nm membrane.

Very recently, STUDDERT and PETERSON (1973) and JOHNSON et al. (1974) corroborated the findings of JOHNSON and CRUICKSHANK and demonstrated particles with a hexagonal outline and an overall diameter of 22 to 24 nm in density gradient fractions associated with FPV/MEV infectivity and hemagglutinin.

3. Physicochemical Characteristics

a) Viral Nucleic Acid and Proteins

The multiplication of FPV/MEV in organs of infected animals and in infected tissue cultures results in the formation of intranuclear basophilic inclusion bodies. Mature homogenous inclusions stained Feulgen-positive and, after treatment with acridine orange, exhibited a brilliant yellow-green colour (MYERS and FRITZ, 1959; JOHNSON and CRUICKSHANK, 1966). Whereas DNase completely abolished Feulgen staining but—unless there was prior treatment with pepsin—only partially removed the acridine orange reaction, application of RNase showed no effect. Finally, the formation of specific inclusions was inhibited by addition of the DNA-antagonist BUdR to the medium of infected cultures (JOHNSON and CRUICKSHANK, 1966; STUDDERT and PETERSON, 1973).

All these data indicated that the nucleic acid of FPV/MEV is of DNA type. Moreover, as JOHNSON and CRUICKSHANK (1966) pointed out, the brilliant green colour after acridine orange staining indicated the presence of double-stranded DNA in intranuclear inclusions. In respect to the configuration of the nucleic acid enclosed in mature virus particles, however, this observation is not conclusive.

The DNA nature of the nucleic acid of the viruses causing feline panleukopenia and mink enteritis have been confirmed by successful labeling of the progeny virus particles with tritiated thymidine (JOHNSON et al., 1974). In addition, both native and denatured nucleic acid molecules extracted from purified virus suspensions sedimented with 23 to 24 S in neutral solutions and at about 16 S in alkaline gradients. Their buoyant density in CsCl was determined to be 1.722 g/ml corresponding to a GC content of 47 per cent. These figures are consistent with the characteristics of a linear single-stranded DNA having a molecular weight of 1.7×10^6 daltons.

The molecular weight of the DNA was calculated to represent 28.5 per cent of a total virus particle weight of 5.9×10^6 daltons. The remaining 71.5 per cent or—in terms of molecular weight—4.2×10^6 daltons, are assumed to represent viral proteins. Electrophoresis of radiolabelled protein on polyacrylamide yielded two polypeptides with molecular weights of 60,300 and 73,100, amounting to 86 and 10 per cent, respectively, of the radioactive amino acids incorporated. A third minor component of molecular weight 39,600 daltons was present at concentration varying between 3 and 6 per cent. Whether the latter polypeptide has to be referred to as a constant constituent of the virion or whether its presence is due to insufficient purification of the particles awaits further clarification (JOHNSON et al., 1974).

b) Buoyant Density

KÄÄRIÄINEN and coworkers (1966), working on MEV, found virus in CsCl density gradient fractions at densities of between 1.30 and 1.33 g/ml. It was noted, however, that centrifugation of virus samples purified by chromatography on DEAE cellulose columns yielded gradients with small amounts of complement-fixing antigen present at 1.38 g/ml. On the other hand, infective FPV extracted from tissue culture harvests by means of Freon treatment showed a maximum density of 1.4 g/ml (STUDDERT and PETERSON, 1973). Infectious virus was also present below the maximum value and since repeated centrifugations did not abolish this banding behaviour, STUDDERT and PETERSON suggested infectious FPV particles to be of rather heterogenous density.

According to JOHNSON and coworkers (1974), the heterogeneity in density is mainly due to the presence of virions containing a varying amount of viral DNA. Analysis based on the density distribution of ^{3}H-thymidine-labelled virus and of viral hemagglutinin indicated that purified tissue culture harvests of both FPV and MEV strains were made up of four particle species with distinct buoyant densities of 1.44, 1.41, 1.36, and 1.31 g/ml. Particles banding around 1.31 g/ml in CsCl could only be detected by hemagglutination and were identified as capsids and breakdown products of capsids devoid of any nucleic acid. Virions recovered from gradient fractions with densities of 1.44 and 1.41 g/ml yielded the complete viral nucleic acid with a molecular weight of 1.7×10^6 daltons, whereas the single-stranded DNA isolated from particles with a buoyant density of 1.36 g/ml had a molecular weight of only 7.8×10^5 daltons. It was assumed that virions concentrating at 1.44 g/ml, whilst having the same DNA as the majority of infectious particles banding at 1.41 g/ml, may have higher densities due to lower protein content or loss of water during aggregate formation.

c) Resistance to Physical and Chemical Agents

In contrast to the early observations of URBAIN (1933) who reported FPV to be a relative labile virus at elevated temperatures, more recent results suggest FPV/MEV to be as resistant to heating as are other parvoviruses. The FAV strain of FPV used by KILHAM and MARGOLIS (1966) to demonstrate the viral etiology of feline ataxia survived heating to 60° C for 30 minutes. JOHNSON (1967) recorded a drop in the infectivity titer from $10^{5.8}$ to $10^{3.4}$ TCID$_{50}$/ml rather than a complete loss of infectivity when MEV and FPV containing tissue culture harvests were held at 75° C for 30 minutes. Moreover, partially purified FPV still proved to be infective after 30 minutes at 80° C (JOHNSON and CRUICKSHANK, 1966).

The high resistance of FPV/MEV is also reflected by the agents' excellent ability to survive storage. Both URBAIN (1933) and SYVERTON et al. (1943) noticed that FPV affected tissues retained their infectivity during storage in 50 per cent glycerol at refrigerator temperature for 35—138 days and MYERS et al. (1959) recorded no loss of titer after keeping infectious organ suspensions for 5 days at 25° C. In addition, FPV harvested from tissue cultures could be stored in Eagle's minimum essential medium at 4° and 25° C for 13 months without any loss of infectivity (POOLE, 1972). At 32° C, however, the titer declined by 2 log$_{10}$ within half a year.

With respect to the effect of chemical agents on the viability of FPV/MEV, it has been found that infectivity of the virus was neither affected by treatment with chloroform or ether nor when the acidity of the virus suspensions was brought to pH 3 (JOHNSON, 1967, 1969; JOHNSON and CRUICKSHANK, 1966; KILHAM and MARGOLIS, 1967; STUDDERT and PETERSON, 1973). In addition, the viruses resisted treatment with trypsin (JOHNSON and CRUICKSHANK, 1966). Formalin, however, at a concentration of 0.5 per cent, was recommended by JOHNSON (1969) as the most effective disinfectant. It should also be remembered that, until successful attempts were made to establish an attenuated FPV strain for vaccination of cats and mink (GORHAM et al., 1965), formalin-inactivated virus derived from organ homogenates or tissue cultures provided an effective vaccine to protect cats against feline panleukopenia and mink against virus enteritis (URBAIN, 1933; GORDON and BELCHER, 1956; WILLS and BELCHER, 1956; MYERS et al., 1959; JOHNSON, 1969).

4. Antigenic Structure and Serological Properties

At present, relatively little information is available on the antigenic structure of FPV/MEV. The inoculation of the virus into susceptible cats and mink regularly induced virus-specific neutralizing antibodies (KIKUTH et al., 1940; LAWRENCE et al., 1943; MYERS et al., 1959; BOLIN, 1957; JOHNSON, 1965) and occasionally low titers of complement-fixing antibodies could be demonstrated. Data concerning the presence of a hemagglutinating antigen, however, are not conclusive. The only agglutination observed with FPV/MEV has been an agglutination of pig erythrocytes at 4° C, characterized by spontaneous elution at room temperature and reoccurrence of agglutination after reincubation in the cold (JOHNSON and CRUICKSHANK, 1966). It is necessary to state that agglutination of pig RBC's by FPV only could be achieved after previous ultrasonication of the virus samples.

Cross neutralization tests in tissue cultures indicated that the infectivity of FPV, MEV, and feline ataxia virus could be neutralized to almost the same degree by both homologous and heterologous antisera (GORHAM *et al.*, 1966; JOHNSON *et al.*, 1967; SCOTT *et al.*, 1970 b) and JOHNSON (1967) has been able to prove the antigenic identity of a standard strain of MEV with six strains of FPV isolated in so clearly separated areas as North America, England, and South Africa. On the basis of the neutralization test, no serologic relationship to members of the hamster-osteolytic viruses (H-1 and RV) could be demonstrated (JOHNSON *et al.*, 1967). Moreover, an antiserum known to protect cats against lethal doses of FPV proved to be ineffective in inhibiting the hemagglutination of various other parvoviruses (HALLAUER *et al.*, 1971) (cf. Table 9, p. 90).

5. Cultivation

a) Host-Cell Range

Since BOLIN in 1957 provided the first evidence for the possibility of cultivating FPV *in vitro* in cells of cat origin, this observation has been confirmed by many investigators. Primary cultures of kitten kidney cells were frequently used (BOLIN, 1957; JOHNSON, 1966; GORHAM *et al.*, 1965, 1966; LUST *et al.*, 1965; KING and CROGHAN, 1965) but cells derived from other cat tissues such as lung, spleen (BOLIN, 1957), heart, diaphragmatic muscle, adrenals, intestine, bone marrow, and mesenteric lymph gland were also shown to be suitable for virus cultivation (JOHNSON, 1966). JOHNSON, however, noticed that a more effective multiplication of FPV takes place in monolayers of heart, diaphragmatic muscle, and adrenal cells than in those of intestinal mucosa and bone marrow, *i.e.* in tissues which are severely damaged *in vivo*.

Although the use of primary kitten kidney cells provides an excellent means to cultivate the virus, there is some risk for explanting tissues already infected *in vivo*, since cats are known to harbour latent FPV infections at a high incidence (cf. section 9). The search for cell cultures of other than cat origin therefore is a necessity. Unfortunately, however, the investigations aimed at this purpose revealed a very limited host cell range of FPV/MEV. In close resemblance to the *in vivo* host range of the viruses, they only multiply in feline, mink, and ferret cells (JOHNSON, 1966), whereas bovine, dog, monkey, or human cells proved to be insusceptible (JOHNSON, 1964). Thus, the only alternative seems to be the use of stable feline cell lines found free of contamination. Attempts pointing into this direction have been made by O'REILLY and WHITAKER (1969) and SCOTT *et al.* (1970a).

b) Cytopathogenicity

In contrast to the observations of BOLIN (1957), who noticed a severe cytopathogenic effect of FPV in primary kitten kidney cell cultures and was able to record infectivity titers as high as $10^{9.5}$ of his tissue culture harvests, more recent studies revealed a quite moderate *in vitro* multiplication and a rather vague cytopathogenic activity of FPV and MEV. The findings of GORHAM *et al.* (1964), LUST *et al.* (1965), JOHNSON (1967a and b), and SCOTT *et al.* (1970a) are well in agreement that in unstained cultures specific CPE is evident as a roughening, thinning, and clumping of the monolayer and may be observed regularly only when virus inocula at concentrations greater than 10^5 TCID$_{50}$/ml are applied. Using highly diluted virus it becomes almost impossible to distinguish a viral

CPE from the effects of ageing of the cell monolayers during the incubation period necessary to allow detectable virus multiplication. To overcome these difficulties in CPE-reading, the staining of infected cultures with either H & E or fluorescein labelled FPV/MEV specific antibodies proved to be valuable (KING and CROGHAN, 1965).

JOHNSON (1965a, b; 1967) especially referred to the occurrence or absence of intranuclear inclusion bodies to determine the infectivity titer of FPV/MEV suspensions in kitten kidney cells. He reported that both the CPE noticeable by mere microscopic observation of unstained cultures and the formation of intranuclear inclusions detectable by H & E staining are transient in nature. Moreover, even after suspensions containing as many as 10^5 $TCID_{50}$ of virus were inoculated under optimal conditions, at no time were more than about 20 per cent of the monolayer's cells affected. The effectiveness of virus multiplication as well as the formation of CPE proved to be closely related to the mitotic index of the infected tissue cultures.

According to JOHNSON, the main features of the cytopathogenic changes detectable by H & E staining of inoculated cell monolayers may be summarized briefly as follows: The first visible effects of virus multiplication become evident in the nucleus as early as 12 hours post inoculation. They consist in an enlargement of the nucleoli, a rarefaction of normal chromatin around the nucleoli and the beginning replacement of normal chromatin by granular eosinophilic material. With progressing time the amount of eosinophilic material increases and, thereby, leads to a distinct margination of the normal chromatin. Already at this stage the inclusion may change colour from eosinophilia towards the deep homogenous basophilia characteristic for mature inclusion bodies. Finally, the basophilic inclusion retracts from the now thickened and dark staining nuclear membrane which then frequently has a wrinkeled and rough appearance. In parallel to these stages of development, the originally basophilic nucleoli enlarge, are dislocated to the nuclear membrane, round off, may become eosinophilic, and then disappear completely. As a final step, the affected nuclei are freed from their surrounding cytoplasm and, thus, give rise to a dark black overlay on the inoculated cell culture. When this characteristic overlay gradually disappears with progressing incubation time, the affected monolayers may be distinguished from uninoculated controls only by a characteristic thinning of the cell sheet rather than by examining the specific cytologic alterations of the infected cells.

c) Virus Multiplication

When primary kitten kidney cell monolayers, about 25 per cent confluent, were inoculated with FPV (JOHNSON, 1967), the first evidence of virus multiplication could be observed as early as 12 hours post inoculation and consisted in the occurrence of immature intranuclear inclusions as well as in a significant rise in titer of cell-associated virus. With a lag of less than 4 hours and parallel to the maturing of inclusion bodies extracellular virus was found in the media. Both cell-associated and cell-free virus finally reached comparable peak titers about 48 hours p.i., when the mitotic activity of the monolayer, being 100 per cent at zero incubation time, had slowed down to 10 per cent. From there upon, the number of inclusions fell rapidly and disappeared between 3 to 4 days later.

Staining of infected monolayers with fluorescein-conjugated antisera did not bring about any new points of view (KING and CROGHAN, 1965; LUST et al., 1965; JOHNSON, 1967). Specific fluorescence became evident in the nuclei for the first time at 16 hours p.i. During the following 20 hours staining of the affected nuclei was excellent but afterwards the disruption of infected cells led to a scattering of fluorescing debris all over the monolayer and, thus, completely obscured the picture.

The close correlation between cessation of mitotic activity and the termination of virus multiplication in inoculated monolayers should need no further comment. Obviously the fully operating nucleic acid and protein synthesizing enzymic apparatus of the cell—as it is activated during cell division—is necessary for successful reproduction of infective FPV. And, in fact, almost all factors found by JOHNSON (1965, 1967) to inhibit or favour FPV/MEV multiplication were shown to stop or to stimulate mitotic activity. Specific inhibition of virus multiplication by some interferon-like substance or an intracellular inhibitor such as the one described by PEREIRA (1960) for adenovirus could be experimentally excluded. On the other hand, actively growing monolayers, i.e. not yet confluent ones, proved to have a pronounced susceptibility whereas resting cell sheets and aged cultures supported virus proliferation only to a very low degree. In the same way, parameters such as supplementation of culture medium and temperature of incubation led to improved FPV multiplication and enhanced CPE if they stimulated the mitotic activity of the cells. With the use of sera of calves, lambs, pigs, horses, dogs, or rabbits to supplement growth media it has been observed that a high proportion of these sera contain some heat stable substance inhibiting multiplication and cytopathogenic activity of FPV/MEV (JOHNSON, 1967). In the presence of such an inhibitory serum up to 3 logs lower titers may be obtained than with a noninhibitory one. The mechanism of action of the inhibitor is not yet completely investigated but the data available from electron microscopy and filtration studies suggest clumping of the virus particles in the presence of inhibitory serum.

6. Pathogenesis

a) Natural Hosts

Until the first noticed outbreaks of mink enteritis between 1947 and 1952 in Canada both epizootologic examinations and experimental investigations led to the conclusion that the natural and only susceptible host of FPV is the domestic cat (URBAIN, 1933; HAMMON and ENDERS, 1939; KIKUTH et al., 1940; LAWRENCE et al., 1943). Now, during the last decade, experimental studies and various occasional isolations of viruses having just the characteristics of FPV suggest a broader range of species susceptibility including members of the families Felidae, Mustelidae, and Procyonidae (JOHNSON, 1969).

In the family Felidae the virus has been isolated from domestic cats, leopards, tigers, lions, and panthers, and from circumstantial observations it seems to be very likely that all members of this family are naturally susceptible. This assumption is especially supported by the high incidence of specific antibodies present in all feline populations. The latter observation may also be the cause for some contradictory results reported by URBAIN (1933) and SCHOFIELD (1949).

Although it was shown by LAWRENCE *et al.* (1943) that successful experimental infection of cats can easily be achieved after oral, intragastric, intranasal, cutaneous, subcutaneous, intraperitoneal, as well as intravenous inoculation of FPV, URBAIN recorded no clinical signs of illness after inoculation of panthers and SCHOFIELD was not able to infect kittens with a MEV strain of FPV.

From the heavy epizootics observed in Canada and Finland it is evident that the mink *(Mustelidae)* is as susceptible to FPV/MEV infection as members of the family *Felidae*. According to SCHOFIELD, however, there are differences in susceptibility between various strains of ranch mink. During the outbreak of mink enteritis in Ontario (1947—1949) he observed a marked resistance of platinums in contrast to the easily affected standard bred strains. Platinums usually showed only transient diarrhea and only about 10 per cent of the affected animals died. On the contrary, mortality rates in stocks of standard mink were around 50 per cent.

A disease with the clinico-pathologic characteristics of feline panleukopenia has also been observed in populations of coatimundi and racoons. The successful isolation of a virus indistinguishable from FPV/MEV from an affected coatimundi now suggests that at least these members of the family *Procyonidae* are naturally susceptible to FPV (JOHNSON, 1968). Successful experimental infection of a racoon has been reported by GORHAM *et al.* (1966).

Table 5. *The Limited Experimental Host Range of FPV/MEV*

Animal	Susceptibility	References
Ferrets, adult	—	98, 222
neonatal	+	107, 128
Mouse	—	243, 264
Rat	—	115, 264
Hamster	—	115
Guinea pig	—	222, 264
Rabbit	—	243, 264
Cottontail rabbit	—	115
Dog, young and adult	—	115, 264
Hedgehog	—	115
Ground squirrel *(Citellus richardsonii* Sabine*)*	—	243
Rhesus monkey	—	115
Canary	—	115
Guinea fowl	—	264
Duck	—	264
Hen	—	264
Embryonated hen's egg	—	243

b) Experimental Hosts

In the decades that have passed since the infective nature of feline panleukopenia was discovered, many attempts have been made to transmit FPV/MEV
experimentally to a great number of laboratory animals. With only one exception—the ferret *(Mustelidae)*—all animals listed in Table 5 proved to be insusceptible. JOHNSON (1966) noticed that, although tissue cultures of ferret origin
supported multiplication of FPV *in vitro*, parenteral infection of adult ferrets only
resulted in the production of antibodies but never in any clinical illness. When
KILHAM and MARGOLIS (1966), however, during investigations of feline ataxia,
were looking for an experimental host to demonstrate the presumably causative
agent, their experience with the hamster-osteolytic viruses made them use neonatal ferrets. The subsequent cooperation of JOHNSON, MARGOLIS, and KILHAM
(1967) then revealed the identity of FAV and FPV/MEV and, besides that, showed
the same neurotropism and affinity of FPV/MEV for dividing cells as had been
found with the osteolytic agents in hamsters. Thus, only during the neonatal
period when the cells of the outer germinal layer of the cerebellum are still in
active mitosis is it possible to induce the typical picture of feline ataxia by inoculating ferrets with either FAV, FPV, or MEV. The other symptoms of feline
panleukopenia, however, cannot be induced in the ferret in the classical forms as
observed in their natural hosts, *i.e.* cats and mink.

7. Clinico-Pathological Features

During the investigation of FPV/MEV infections, many different names—
feline enteritis, mink enteritis, feline agranulocytosis, feline aleukocytosis, feline
panleukopenia, feline ataxia—have been proposed to characterize the disease induced by these agents in their natural hosts. This nomenclature, of course, frequently gave rise to the question whether all authors were really dealing with
one and the same virus. Thorough experimental animal studies conducted in recent years as well as the extensive work of JOHNSON on the multiplication behaviour of FPV/MEV in tissue culture cells have now provided a key to the explanation of natural infections. The above cited names stand for different syndromes
of a disease and, depending on circumstantial factors such as age of the animal,
mode of infection, and possible presence of other infective agents, a certain syndrome may become more obvious than the others in the course of the illness. In
all cases, however, the pathogenic action of FPV/MEV is based on its predilection
for actively growing cells.

a) Classical Disease

Considering the infection of susceptible animals older than 9 days, a stage of
development at which, in felines at least, active growth of the cerebellar cortical
cells ceases, FPV/MEV infection of both felines and mink usually is characterized
by a mean incubation period of 6 days. During natural as well as experimental
infections, however, this period may vary between 2 and 10 days (SYVERTON
et al., 1943; LUCAS and RISER, 1945; SCHOFIELD, 1949; BENTINCK-SMITH, 1949;
JOHNSON, 1965, 1969; ROHOVSKY and GRIESEMER, 1967).

(1) *Felines*

The onset of acute disease in felines frequently is indicated by mild pyrexia accompanied by listlessness and inappetence of the animal. Extremely elevated body temperatures usually can only be recorded in the following 24 hours, when vomiting of food, anorexia, depression, and dehydration become evident for the first time. With progressing disease these symptoms become more pronounced and may also be associated with diarrhea. However, vomiting, diarrhea, as well as nasal and ocular discharge occur most irregular and presumably depend on simultaneous infection of the animal by other viruses. In fact, BITTLE *et al.* (1961) were able to produce the classical syndrome including vomiting, pyrexia, diarrhea, and dehydration regularly only by simultaneous infection of cats with FPV and a myxovirus isolated by BOLIN (1957) from FPV-infected tissue cultures. Overt disease characterized in this way, usually lasts for 2 to 4 days and during this time, according to JOHNSON (1969), the cat assumes "a typical pan-leukopenia attitude, crouched with head between paws".

In parallel to the initial slow rise in temperature, a gradual fall in total white blood cell (WBC) counts may be observed towards the end of the incubation period (JOHNSON, 1965). Detailed studies revealed, however, that lymphocytes and neutrophiles are especially reduced. The height of clinical disease also coincides with the appearance of the lowest WBC counts and, in some respect, the figures recorded are directly related to the severity of the disease. It has been said that illness becomes overt when counts of neutrophiles and lymphocytes fall short of 7,000 cells per c.mm. In severe cases usually less than 1,000 cells per c.mm are present.

Following the experimental observations and the argumentations of HAMMON and ENDERS (1939b), KIKUTH *et al.* (1940), LAWRENCE *et al.* (1943), LUCAS and RISER (1945), and JOHNSON (1969), the cause of this reduction in WBC counts has to be looked upon as being the primary and direct attack of FPV upon the lymphoid tissues and blood forming organs. Soon after infection the initial response in the lymph nodes consists in a draining off of lymphocytes from medullary spaces and cords accompanied by severe phagocytosis of erythrocytes. Typical intranuclear inclusions have been found in the tissues as early as 3 days after infection and destruction of stem cells and lymphoblasts may finally result in lymphopenia. When the virus reaches the bone marrow, presumably via the blood stream, the appearance of similar inclusion bodies in the primitive blood cells suggests the very same specific attack and, thus, infection may lead to neutropenia.

In parallel with the destruction of lymphoid and blood-forming tissues due to the multiplication of FPV in the intestinal lymph nodes and lymphoid tissues, invasion of the gastrointestinal mucosa occurs. Thereby, especially in the terminal portion of the small intestine and in the duodenum, extensive destruction of villi and of the epithelium of the crypts of Lieberkühn results. The presence of typical "ballooned" cells and those containing eosinophilic to basophilic staining intranuclear inclusions in the crypts is a common finding.

True secondary reactions are restricted to liver, kidneys, and pancreas. These organs usually respond late in disease but the resulting damage may be greater than that found in the primary centers. Spleen, liver, and kidney also offer the best source for reisolation of virus and recent tissue culture studies suggest that in kidneys of recovered animals infectious virus might persist for a long time despite an impressive immunity (SIZA et al., 1971).

In fully susceptible cats, i.e. in those without any protective immunity, termination of the disease either by death or more or less rapid recovery is not necessarily linked to the severity of tissue destruction but mainly to the condition of the animal at the time infection took place. Death may intervene at any stage of the disease following the initial high temperature response; usually, however, it occurs after 2 to 4 days of manifest illness. Revocery, on the other hand, at the same time is signalled by a detectable rise in WBC counts and the appearance of antibodies. Although dehydration and listlessness of the cat may disappear within a few days, it frequently takes the recovered animal several weeks to regain normal body weight and many also may suffer from chronic diarrhea.

(2) Mink

Whereas many features of FPV/MEV infection in mink such as incubation period, duration of acute illness, temperature response, anorexia, dehydration, apathic behaviour, and typical posture of the animal are almost exactly the same as in felines, the outstanding characteristic of the disease in this species is the most regular occurrence of a severe enteritis (SCHOFIELD, 1949; WILLS, 1952; GORHAM and HARTSOUGH, 1954; MYERS et al., 1959; REYNOLDS, 1969). Peracute infections in which anorexia is followed by death in 12 to 24 hours without any evidence of diarrhea (KNOX, 1960) are not found frequently.

Towards the end of the incubation period, i.e. 4—6 days after infection, onset of disease is indicated by the appearance of soft, watery stools containing greyish-white, sometimes bloodstained mucus. During the following 24 hours, parallel to a rise in temperature, the feces then contain the highest observable amount of intestinal casts which usually are almost wholly composed of fibrin, tenacious mucus and desquamated epithelium. If vomiting occurs, the vomitus also may consist of a yellowish, watery fluid admixed with small quantities of clear mucus. Whereas anorexia and dehydration are more pronounced with progressing disease, the stools are found to become excessively fluid and almost devoid of mucus. As a rule, normally formed feces reappear after 5 to 6 days onset of acute illness. If MEV infection in mink is associated with manifest enteritis, especially in kits, mortality rates up to 80 per cent may be recorded.

Necropsy of animals having died at the height of disease or shortly after the crisis had passed revealed intestines containing a hemorrhagic catarrhal exudate, congested mesenteric lymph nodes, and dark enlarged spleen with hemorrhages just beneath the capsule. Histopathologic examinations of the intestines suggested the hemorrhagic content of the gut and the casts being due to marked necrosis and desquamation of the columnar epithelium of the intestinal mucosa. Comparable to the finding in affected felines, the crypts of Lieberkühn harboured "ballooned" epithelial cells and those with typical intranuclear inclusions.

Several investigators also reported a frequent reduction in WBC counts accompanying the overt signs of mink enteritis (MACPHERSON, 1956; MYERS et al., 1959; BURGER and GORHAM, 1960). The significance and diagnostic value of these observations were unknown for a long time due to controversies on the normal blood picture of mink. Only in a recent paper REYNOLDS (1969) showed that

WBC counts in normal mink may range from 6,100 to 13,000 cells per c.mm and infected animals, with total counts less than 5,000 cells per c.mm can be considered to be leukopenic. Evaluating the results of the above mentioned authors with this scale, about 60 to 80 per cent of the affected mink would have developed clear leukopenia between the fifth and the tenth day following infection. Leukopenia largely has to be attributed to a decrease in circulating lymphocytes and only secondly to an evident, however less marked, loss of neutrophils. This observation is only in part compatible with the hematologic changes in FPV affected cats.

b) Ataxia

In the introduction to the clinicopathologic section (p. 61) it has been pointed out that the syndromes induced by FPV/MEV infection in susceptible species may depend on circumstantial factors to which the age of the animal and the mode of infection also belong. In the genesis of classical FPV/MEV disease these two parameters are of only limited importance; however, in the case of the ataxic syndrome of kittens both are of outstanding significance. KILHAM and MARGOLIS (1966) as well as JOHNSON et al. (1967) clearly showed that in analogy to the ataxia produced by the osteolytic viruses in hamsters, the ataxia of kittens originates from a selective attack on the outer germinal layer of the cerebellum in unborn or neonate kittens by FPV/MEV. Since multiplication of the virus depends on the availability of cells in active mitosis, the possibility for this attack and, thus, for the neurologic manifestation of FPV/MEV infection, exists only in the short time until about nine days after birth, after which time the cerebellum of felines has gained its definite stage of development. The cerebellar hypoplasia resulting from the destruction of the cells of the outer germinal layer during this time space turns into manifest ataxia when 3 to 4 weeks after birth the infected kittens become active and move around. The animals may then show a coarse tremor, walk with a wide base and fall repeatedly. In natural infections usually the whole litter is affected. The original FAV strain isolated by KILHAM and MARGOLIS, as well as FPV/MEV reference strains, lead to the same histopathologic changes and clinical manifestation whether inoculated intracerebrally into newborn kittens or ferrets. For experimental studies, however, ferrets should be preferred, since this species has no natural susceptibility for FPV/MEV and, hence, no specific antibodies passively transmitted from the mothers to their offspring will interfere with infection. Another interesting difference between both species consists in the fact that in kittens—the natural host—infection spreads spontaneously within a litter from inoculated animals to uninoculated controls whereas control ferrets regularly remain unaffected. Experimentally inoculated, spontaneously, and naturally infected kittens, besides the cerebellar injury and the development of overt ataxia, in general show no other signs of disease. It seems, therefore, that at this age of the animals, the rapidly dividing cells of the cerebellum in the external germinal layer are the only target of FPV/MEV infection.

Histopathologic examination of the cerebellum of infected animals revealed typical intranuclear inclusions in the dividing cells of the outer germinal layer. Lysis of this affected cell population finally resulted in the hypoplastic state of the cerebellum, characterized by the virtual absence of a definitive granular cortex. Although less pronounced and sometimes delayed in appearance, specific destruction of Purkinje cells was evident. In this cell type typical alterations mainly consisted in vesicularization of the nuclei and vacuolization within the cytoplasm. Complete destruction of affected Purkinje cells may result; however, at no phase of affection could inclusion bodies be found.

Circumstantial evidence already showed that FPV/MEV is able to pass the placental barrier of pregnant queens and, therefore, most of the observed cases of ataxia in kittens are assumed to be acquired by *in utero* infections. The studies of KILHAM and MARGOLIS (1966), and KILHAM et al. (1967) strongly support this assumption. *In utero* inoculation of foetuses at about the midst of gestation finally resulted in the delivery of kittens with pronounced ataxia and, following necropsy, severe cerebellar hypoplasia could be observed. This mode of infection, however, resulted in the frequent finding of resorption of the foetuses, mummification, stillbirth, abortions, and neonatal death.

8. Immunity

Depending on the reduction of the amount of actively growing cells with progressive maturation of tissues, older animals of the natural susceptible hosts of FPV/MEV may only show a very limited spectrum of clinical reactions following infection and, hence, exhibit a certain age-related resistance to the virus. Without the development of an actively acquired immunity, however, resistance to FPV/MEV is never a complete one (LAWRENCE et al., 1943; WILLS and BELCHER, 1956). The relationship between the presence of neutralizing antibodies to FPV/MEV in the serum of cats and the severity of the symptoms in these animals after challenge infection with FPV became evident when *in vitro* neutralization tests were performed to select susceptible cats for vaccine tests. KING and CROGHAN (1965) thereby stated that all animals having antibody titers higher than 1:2 would show nothing other than signs of anorexia 5 to 7 days after infection and would then recover quickly. Immune kittens with antibody levels of 1:250 and 1:325 before inoculation developed neither leokopenia nor any clinical response at all (JOHNSON, 1965).

The development of an attenuated tissue culture live vaccine made it possible to follow the formation of FPV antibodies in infected animals (GORHAM et al., 1965, 1966). In cat sera detectable amounts of neutralizing FPV antibodies were found as early as 8 days post infection, whereas in minks noticeable antibody production already occurred after 3 days. Fifteen days after inoculation titers between 1:16 and 1:60 could be recorded and after 30 days the serum of cats neutralized 100 $TCID_{50}$ even at dilutions of about 1:150. These results are well in accordance with observations obtained from cats suffering from acute experimentally induced leukopenia. Recovery from the acute phase of illness coincided with the production of specific antibody and 4 weeks p.i. S/N antibody titers of 1:175—1:340 could be measured (JOHNSON, 1965).

Under natural conditions, antibody levels found in members of feline populations were lower (1:5—1:120), but were present at a high incidence (about 70 per cent) (JOHNSON, 1965). These data account for passive immunity of kittens as well as for active immunity of adult animals. Depending on the immune status of the queens, passively transmitted neutralizing antibodies persist in suckling

kittens for 3—12 weeks (JOHNSON, 1965; SCOTT et al., 1970). From this age on-
ward, the development of active immunity can be followed. In such cases JOHN-
SON assumed the active formation of FPV/MEV antibodies to be due to infections at the subclinical level. Since, as with the hamster-osteolytic agents and
PPV, infective FPV/MEV was recovered from tissues of immune animals, feline
as well as mink populations presumably harbour a high percentage of virus carriers from which the agent is transmitted to the so far uninfected immature animals (O'REILLY, 1969; CSIZA et al., 1971; BOUILLANT and HANSON, 1965;
GORHAM and HARTSOUGH, 1955).

9. Epizootiology

Whereas during the first decades of this century fulminating epizootics of
feline panleukopenia have been reported in Europe (VERGE and CHRISTOFERONI,
1928; URBAIN, 1933), North America (LAWRENCE and SYVERTON, 1938; HAMMON
and ENDERS, 1939), and Brazil (MACHIAVELLO and BEZERRA COUTINHO, 1940),
there is much evidence suggesting that this classical infectious disease of felines is
no longer of such outstanding importance. In more recent times FPV/MEV infections on a comparably large scale have only been observed in colonies of
ranch mink (SCHOFIELD, 1949; WILLS, 1952) and outbreaks of feline panleukopenia
with a morbidity up to 100 per cent are usually restricted to feline population of
isolated communities such as farms and villages (JOHNSON, 1959) where neither
vaccination nor natural infections have given rise to a sufficient active immunity.
In town cats, however, about 70 per cent of the animals are efficiently protected
and natural infections, originating presumably from carrier animals, in general
only occur at the subclinical level.

When fully susceptible populations of cats or mink were affected by FPV/MEV,
the disease induced by this agent proved to be highly contagious. HAMMON and
ENDERS (1939), KIKUTH et al. (1940), and LAWRENCE et al. (1943) were unable to
prevent animals from contracting the disease when cats were kept in the usual
animal quarters. During the first recognized outbreaks of mink enteritis in Canada
a very similar rapid dissemination of the virus within the animal stock of affected farms and from ranch to ranch was observed (SCHOFIELD, 1949; WILLS,
1952). One of the main reasons for this pronounced infectivity may surely be
found in the extreme stability of the causative agent allowing it even to survive
under unfavourable conditions. Other factors contributing to the spread of the
disease are the regular presence of infective virus in feces, urine, nasal secretions
and saliva of affected animals during acute illness (URBAIN, 1933; LAWRENCE et
al., 1943; SCHOFIELD, 1949).

According to the latter observations, transmission of FPV/MEV by contact,
by nasal droplets and via contaminated food appears to be the most likely means.
The significance of the gastrointestinal and the respiratory routes as natural por-
tals of entry has been supported by the results of LAWRENCE et al. (1943) and
REYNOLDS (1969) who clearly showed that cats and mink infected by mouth or
stomach tube, and cats infected intranasally readily developed the full spectrum
of clinical disease within the usual incubation period. Finally, the role of fleas and
other insects feeding upon sick animals in the transfer of the virus to susceptible

cats and mink must be drawn in account since infective FPV/MEV is present in the blood stream of both species during the incubation period and during the acute phase of disease and intravenous as well as cutaneous infection of the animal also proved to be possible.

Discussing the epizootiologic characteristics of FPV/MEV infections, special reference must be made to the fact that affected animals may excrete virus for several months following recovery. GORHAM and HARTSOUGH (1955) already deduced the probability of such carriers from the regular reappearance of mink enteritis in successive kit crops and there is also strong circumstantial evidence that a low percentage of cats suffering from infectious cerebellar ataxia or having recovered from panleukopenia shed the virus (KILHAM and MARGOLIS, 1966; JOHNSON, 1969). In addition, O'REILLY and WHITAKER (1969) were able to isolate FPV out of tissue cultures established from kidney cortices of apparently healthy cats. This observation is in line with the persistence of the osteolytic viruses in tissues of immune rats and hamsters (see chapter A) and the presence of PPV in kidney cells of immune pigs (see chapter C). From the latter virus/host systems it is not exactly known whether affected animals regularly excrete virus; however, evidence has been provided that the apparently delicate equilibrium between virus present in the organs of rats and active immunity of the animal can easily be disturbed by circumstantial factors and, hence, disease may become overt. Assuming a similar possibility for the FPV/cat and MEV/mink systems, almost all animals whether latently infected or recovered from clinical disease have to be considered to form a huge virus reservoir.

E. Bovine Parvovirus (BPV)

1. History

In 1961 ABINANTI and WARFIELD recovered a virus from the intestinal tract of normal calves which showed several features not in accordance with any of the then known viruses. The size of the particle was estimated to be approximately 30 nm. It multiplied in bovine embryonic kidney cell cultures and there induced the formation of a vague but progressive CPE. Of outstanding importance, however, appeared the ability of the virus to agglutinate red blood cells of human and guinea pig origin as well as the fact that the very same erythrocytes adsorbed readily to infected cells. ABINANTI and WARFIELD therefore referred to the newly isolated agent as to the hemadsorbing enteric (HADEN) virus of calves.

Further attempts to characterize the virus particle (SPAHN et al., 1966) yielded results suggesting the nucleic acid to be of RNA type. In consequence, HADEN virus was classified within the enterovirus group. More recently, however, reliable information has accumulated (STORZ and WARREN, 1970; BACHMANN, 1971) justifying the classification of HADEN virus as bovine parvovirus 1 into the parvovirus group.

The parvoviruses isolated so far from cattle in the United States, Europe, and North Africa were serologically indistinguishable from the original HADEN strain. Isolates recovered in Japan shared similar characteristics. One single strain, however, was reported to be serologically unrelated (INABA et al., 1973) and, hence, has been proposed to represent a second type of bovine parvovirus.

2. Size of the Particle and Physicochemical Properties

It was shown that partially purified tissue culture harvests of bovine parvo-viruses can be passaged through filters with a pore size of 50 nm without a significant loss of infectivity (ABINANTI and WARFIELD, 1961; BACHMANN, 1971; VINCENT, 1971; INABA et al., 1973a, b). Moreover, electron microscopy of concentrated virus samples and of density gradient fractions revealed spherical, envelopeless particles with a mean diameter of 20 to 23 nm (BACHMANN, 1971; HOGGAN, 1971; STORZ and BATES, 1973; INABA et al., 1973a, b). These observations are in excellent agreement with the diameter of 18—20 nm reported for intranuclear spherical structures detected in ultrathin sections of HADEN virus infected calf kidney cells (VINCENT, 1971; STORZ and BATES, 1973). Data concerning the symmetry of the particle, however, are so far not available.

JOHNSON and HOGGAN (1973) have analyzed the proteins of purified parvovirus 1 in neutral SDS-polyacrylamide gels. They found three different types of polypeptides. The major one had a molecular weight of 67,000 and accounted for 73—83 per cent of total virion protein. The two minor components showed molecular weights of 77,000 and 85,500 and were present in an amount of 7.7—10.6 and 9.6—13.8 per cent, respectively. As could be shown by means of indirect methods (inhibition of virus multiplication by IUdR, BUdR, as well as by actionmycine D) (STORZ and WARREN, 1970; BACHMANN, 1971; INABA et al., 1973a, b; STORZ and BATES, 1973), these proteins enclose a nucleic acid of DNA-type.

Tissue culture harvests of bovine parvovirus 1 usually contained three to four particle species which more or less readily could be separated by buoyant density centrifugation in CsCl gradients: A small fraction banding at densities around 1.41 g/ml, hemagglutinating, infectious virions at 1.38—1.41 g/ml, and merely hemagglutinating particles accumulating around 1.35 as well as at 1.31 g/ml (BACHMANN, 1971; JOHNSON and HOGGAN, 1973; INABA et al., 1973b). According to sedimentation studies in sucrose gradients and to electron microscopic observations, the hemagglutinating particles recovered from gradient fractions with densities of 1.31 g/ml appeared to be viral capsids devoid of nucleic acid.

Like all the other members of the genus parvovirus, bovine parvovirus is of outstanding stability. It withstands heating to 56° C and to 60° C for six hours without an appreciable loss of infectivity (ABINANTI and WARFIELD, 1961; BACHMANN, 1971; STORZ and BATES, 1973; INABA et al., 1973a, b) and heating to 70° C for a period of two hours resulted in a reduction of the infectivity titer of two $\log_{10}$ only. In addition, changing the pH between 3 and 8 remained without effect on viral infectivity and no loss in viability could be recorded after treating viral suspensions with ether, chloroform, sodium dodecylsulphate, 1 M $MgCl_2$, and 1 per cent trypsin.

3. Antigenicity

Bovine parvovirus has been found to agglutinate erythrocytes of several species. Most consistent results could be obtained using guinea pig and human group 0 red blood cells (BACHMANN, 1971; INABA et al., 1973a; STORZ and BATES, 1973), but erythrocytes of dog (BACHMANN, 1971), horse, sheep, goat, hamster, duck, goose (INABA et al., 1973a), and of rat origin (BATES et al., 1972) were also found suitable. No agglutination has been observed using bovine, rabbit, cat, mouse, and chicken RBC's (BACHMANN, 1971; INABA et al., 1973a; STORZ and BATES, 1973). Agglutination occurred both at 4° and 25° C, yet, titers read at 25° C were usually lower than those obtained at refrigerator temperature (BACHMANN, 1971; BATES et al., 1972; INABA et al., 1973a). Neither at 25° nor at 4° C was the reaction followed by spontaneous elution of the virus.

According to extensive hemagglutination-inhibition testing, all bovine parvoviruses isolated in the United States, Europe, and North Africa, as well as the majority of the strains recovered in Japan are of identical antigenicity. Virusneutralization tests supported this observation and in bovine kidney cell cultures infected with ten different isolates, viral antigen could be readily detected in infected cells by means of staining with fluorescent antibody prepared against a reference strain of bovine parvovirus 1 (BATES et al., 1972). At present, the only strain of bovine parvovirus antigenically distinguishable from the original HADEN-strain has been isolated in Japan (INABA et al., 1973b). The latter strain obviously shares only a minor antigenic component in common with the original strain of bovine parvovirus.

For bovine parvovirus 1 it could be shown that there is no serologic relationship to RV, H-1, MVM, FPV, PPV (BACHMANN, 1971), as well as to TVX, LuIII, and RTV (HALLAUER et al., 1971). No data, however, are available so far concerning the antigenic relatedness of bovine parvovirus type 2 to the other known parvoviruses.

4. Cultivation

ABINANTI and WARFIELD (1961) recovered the original HADEN-strain of bovine parvovirus from bovine embryonic kidney cell cultures inoculated with fecal specimens of calves. In this culture system the virus grew to levels of 10^5 $TCID_{50}/ml$ whereas rhesus monkey kidney tissue cultures inoculated simultaneously did not support viral replication.

Since that original report a variety of primary bovine cell cultures has been found suitable for both isolation and cultivation of bovine parvovirus. In general, primary bovine kidney and testicle cells were used successfully (BACHMANN, 1971; VINCENT, 1971; INABA et al., 1973a). As STORZ and BATES (1973) noted however, virus isolated following infection of actively growing primary cells of bovine fetal lung, spleen, testicle, and adrenal gland origin showed higher infectivity and hemagglutinating titers than virus harvested from bovine fetal kidney cells. In the hands of the same investigators the virus did not multiply in established cell lines of bovine, monkey, mouse, hamster, and human origin and only abortive infection with gradual loss of infectivity could be observed following inoculation of bovine parvovirus into primary cell cultures derived from chicken and guinea pig embryos (STORZ and BATES, 1973; BATES and STORZ, 1973).

Depending on the dose of virus applied and the mitotic index of the inoculated cell culture, multiplication of bovine parvovirus 1 in susceptible cells is paralleled by appearance of cytopathologic changes 3 to 7 days following infection. Such a CPE is characterized by granulation, rounding off, and finally by disintegration of infected cells. Moreover, H & E staining may reveal eosinophilic to basophilic intranuclear inclusion bodies developing as early as 18 to 24 hours after infection (BACHMANN, 1971; VINCENT, 1971; BATES *et al.*, 1972; INABA *et al.*, 1973a) and suggesting the nucleus to be the main site of virus replication. The latter assumption is consistent with results of ultrahistological studies (VINCENT, 1971; STORZ and BATES, 1973)* demonstrating the presence of large numbers of empty capsids and electron dense spherical particles about 18—22 nm in size in nuclei of infected cells. Intranuclear location was also ascertained by means of immunofluorescence tests (BATES and STORZ, 1973).

So far, the growth cycle of bovine parvovirus has been studied in randomly growing cell cultures only*. Using actively growing bovine fetal lung cells infected at a multiplicity of 6 plaque-forming units per cell, STORZ and BATES (1973) observed a lag period of 16 hours until a significant amount of hemagglutinating and infectious progeny virus could be detected intracellularly. Cell-associated virus then increased logarithmically up to 48 hours post infection. On the other hand, extracellular virus could not be demonstrated before 30 hours p.i. and maximum amounts were present in the culture medium at 60 hours p.i. At any time, however, titers of cell-free virus were consistently lower than those recorded for cell-associated bovine parvovirus.

5. Pathogenicity

According to the results of several serologic surveys, bovine parvovirus 1 is broadly distributed in cattle. ABINANTI and WARFIELD (1961) measured hemagglutination-inhibiting antibody titers of 1:20 or greater in 86 per cent of sera of adult cattle and similar results have been obtained by SPAHN *et al.* (1966), VINCENT (1971), STORZ *et al.* (1972), and STORZ and BATES (1973). When sera of species other than bovines were tested for their potency to inhibit hemagglutination of bovine parvovirus, relatively high inhibition titers have been recorded with sera of cynomolgus monkeys and guinea pigs, lower titers were present in sera of dogs, goats, and horses, whereas serum of sheep never showed any inhibitory action (STORZ *et al.*, 1972). The real meaning of these results, however, is not clear since the authors made no reference as to whether or not the titers observed could be influenced or even abolished by pretreatment of the sera with kaolin or by other techniques capable of removing unspecific inhibitors.

Up to date bovine parvovirus 1 has usually been isolated from fecal samples of calves most of which experienced enteric disease (ABINANTI and WARFIELD, 1961; VINCENT, 1971; BATES *et al.*, 1972; INABA *et al.*, 1973a). Attempts to isolate a parvovirus from 49 specimens from calves that were aborted or that died neonatally, as well as from calves with cerebellar or cerebral hypoplasia or from calves with corticocerebral necrosis were unsuccessful (JOHNSON, 1969). STORZ and BATES (1973) suggested that this failure as well as the relatively small number of positive isolations from fecal specimens might be attributed to the use of insensitive cell cultures and to the use of bovine sera containing small amounts of specific antibodies to supplement culture media.

The disease-inducing potential of bovine parvovirus has not been completely assessed. In a study reported by BATES *et al.* (1972) viruses could be isolated from 33 out of 129 fecal and intestinal samples of calves suffering from diarrhea du-

---

* See addendum.

ring the first week after birth. Most of these viruses were enteroviruses and only ten isolates could be classified as parvoviruses. Calves that recovered showed rising antibody titers against bovine parvovirus. The presence of antibodies, however, did not exclude shedding of the parvovirus within the feces. As STORZ and BATES noted in a more recent paper (1973) surviving calves in one herd were retarded in their growth and appeared stunted.

Experimental infection of colostrum-deprived calves and of calves receiving colostrum free of parvovirus antibody resulted in the development of diarrhea within 24 to 48 hours independent of whether the animals were inoculated orally or intravenously (STORZ and BATES, 1973). Initially the diarrhea was mucoid but later on it became watery. Virus was excreted in the feces from the time diarrhea became apparent onto the end of the experiment at 11 days after inoculation. Both by means of reisolation and by immunofluorescent staining it could be demonstrated that intestinal cells at all levels of the intestinal tract became infected, yet, the small intestine was infected most heavily. Besides that, virus was present in lymph nodes, spleen, thymus, kidney, lung, adrenal gland, ovaries, testicles, heart muscle, cerebrospinal fluid, the brain stem, and the cerebellum. Such a massive invasion of almost all tissues may result from the development of an extensive viremia. After oral inoculation virus could be recovered from the leukocyte fraction of blood samples as early as 48 hours p.i. and, following infection by the intravenous route, viremia lasted for 4 to 6 days.

F. Minute Virus of Canines (MVC)

In 1967 BINN and coworkers reported the isolation of a small virus from the feces of asymptomatic dogs. The particle characteristics listed in a more recent paper (BINN et al., 1970) suggest a membership of this agent in the parvovirus group.

According to electron microscopic and filtration studies, the virus is about 20—21 nm in size. After equilibrium centrifugation, the hemagglutinating and, in a permanent cell line of dog origin, cytopathogenic agent was found to accumulate at a density of 1.4 g/ml. The virus resisted the treatment with ether, chloroform, heat (60° C, 1 hour), and incubation at pH 3. The DNA nature of viral nucleic acid was assessed on the basis of inhibition of virus multiplication by means of 5-iodo-deoxyuridine and the development of intranuclear inclusion bodies which stained brightly green following acridine orange staining.

Agglutination of red blood cells proved restricted to rhesus or African green monkey erythrocytes. The reaction took place only at 5° C. No agglutination could be observed with guinea pig, human 0, dog, goose, rat, sheep, bovine, and pig erythrocytes at 5°, 25°, or 37° C. Hemagglutination inhibition tests revealed no serologic relationship of the minute virus of canines to H-1, MVM, RV (BINN et al., 1970), FPV, PPV, RTV, TVX, and LuIII-virus (SIEGL et al., unpublished).

The pathogenic potency of the virus is unknown; however, due to the high incidence of specific HI-antibodies in dog sera (70 per cent) the minute virus of canines is apparently wide spread in dog populations.

G. Parvoviruses Isolated from Permanent Human Cell Lines

1. History

When HALLAUER and KRONAUER (1960), engaged in *in vitro* studies of yellow fever virus (YFV), succeeded in extraction of YFV-specific hemagglutinin by means of an alkaline buffer without damage of the cell cultures, they introduced a very sensitive method for becoming aware of latent parvoviruses present in cultured cells. HALLAUER and KRONAUER encountered this special problem when uninfected control cultures subjected to the extraction procedure also yielded an infective hemagglutinating agent, its features, however, being distinct from YFV (HALLAUER and KRONAUER, 1962). Preliminary electron microscopy of extracts showed that the hemagglutinating property was apparently associated with spherical particles about 30 nm in diameter (ZWILLENBERG and HALLAUER, 1962). A subsequent, more thorough study concerning the morphology as well as the physicochemical and biological properties of the hemagglutinating isolates HALLAUER and KRONAUER (1966/67, unpublished results) then furnished sufficient evidence for classifying the viruses within the picodna(parvo-)virus group established by MAYOR and MELNICK in 1966.

Between 1960 and 1971 43 permanent human cell strains collected from 19 almost exclusively European laboratories were tested for the presence of the small hemagglutinating viruses (HALLAUER *et al.*, 1971). 38 successful isolations were made and the isolates could be grouped into three distinct serotypes represented by virus strains KBSH, TVX, and LuIII. The biological and physicochemical characteristics of these reference strains were in conformity with the requirements for membership within the parvovirus group (HALLAUER *et al.*, 1971, 1972; SIEGL *et al.*, 1971). At present, however, the most pertinent problem arising from these studies, *i.e.* the origin of the tissue culture contaminants and the means by which they have been introduced into the cultures, is still a matter of discussion. For two of the serotypes, all attempts to trace the natural host have failed. Only reference strain KBSH was shown to be closely related to or even identical with porcine parvovirus. Circumstantial evidence (HALLAUER *et al.*, 1971) and recently reported direct isolations (CROGHAN *et al.*, 1973) suggested that viruses belonging to this serotype have been transmitted to the cultures by the use of trypsin derived from the pancreas of PPV infected pigs.

2. Morphology

The morphological features of the virus particles found in density gradient purified preparations of selected reference strains were all in accordance with the characteristics reported for other parvoviruses (SIEGL *et al.*, 1971). After negative staining the spherical particles proved to be devoid of an envelope and the overall diameter of the individual viruses ranged from 17 to 29 nm. However, a graphic summation of the size distribution of the tested virus strains showed that the majority of the particles measured 19—21 nm in diameter.

From viruses into which the stain had penetrated the size of the core was estimated to be 14—17 nm. At the periphery of some few particles as many as 7—10 distinct subunits could be counted and reverse printing of electron micrographs occasionally revealed capsomeres in either five- or six-fold symmetrical arrangement. It was concluded from these observations that, in good agreement with the suggestion of VASQUEZ and BRAILOVSKY (1965) for Kilham rat virus (RV), 32 discrete capsomeres about 30 Å in diameter are arranged in the capsid according to the symmetrical requirements of a pentakis dodecahedron.

3. Physicochemical Characteristics

a) Type and Configuration of Nucleic Acid

First evidence concerning type and configuration of the nucleic acid of the isolated viruses has been obtained by means of indirect methods. Both infectivity and hemagglutinin production were suppressed in tissue cultures by treatment with 5-iodo-deoxyuridine (IUdR) at a concentration of 100 μg/ml. The inhibitory action of the IUdR could be readily reversed by addition of 24 μg/ml thymidine. It was concluded, therefore, that the nucleic acid of the viruses is of DNA type (SIEGL, et al., 1971).

For further discrimination between RNA and DNA and, moreover, between double-stranded or single-stranded DNA, highly concentrated and purified droplet preparations of strains KBSH, TVX, and LuIII were stained with acridine orange according to MAYOR and DIWAN (1961) and MAYOR and HILL (1961). Dried droplets of the tested viruses exhibited a redish fluorescence being either indicative for RNA or for single-stranded DNA. Since, however, this specific staining was absent after digesting the preparations with DNase but never after treatment with RNase, the nucleic acid was supposed to be DNA of single-stranded configuration.

For both KBSH- and LuIII-virus the assumed DNA-nature and single-stranded configuration of the nucleic acid have been confirmed by direct analysis of the isolated molecules (SIEGL, 1972, 1973). The nucleic acid contained in complete as well as in "incomplete" virus particles (for definition see section 3 c) could be readily labelled with radioactive thymidine. The DNA extracted from infectious particles sedimented with about 24 S at neutral pH whether native, denatured at pH 13 followed by neutralization, or denaturation at 100° C. Coefficients recorded during sedimentation in alkaline solution for KBSH- and LuIII-virus DNA were 18.3 and 16 S, respectively. Both DNA's banded in CsCl at the rather high density of 1.724 g/ml. According to RIVA et al. (1969), a single-stranded DNA having such a buoyancy behaviour should contain about 48 per cent guanine and cytosine.

For DNA isolated from infectious particles of LuIII-virus the single-stranded configuration of the molecule could be ascertained by complete elution from benzoylated-naphtoylated-DEAE cellulose columns under conditions yielding only single-stranded DNA. Moreover, the nucleic acid was readily digested by the single-strand specific exonuclease of the sponge *Verongia aerophoba* and electron microcsopy revealed kinked linear molecules about 1.6 μ in length. From all these data it was finally concluded that KBSH- as well as LuIII-virus contain a linear single-stranded DNA with a molecular weight of between 1.4 to 1.6 × 10⁶ daltons. This DNA constitutes 26.5 to 28 per cent of the total molecular weight of an infectious virus particle.

The nucleic acid molecules extracted from the so-called incomplete virus particles which banded at 1.34 to 1.36 g/ml in CsCl formed a very heterogenous population as far as the molecular weight is concerned. The invariance of the sedimentation characteristics of the molecules at neutral pH after denaturation as well as a buoyant density of 1.724 g/ml in CsCl nevertheless suggest a single-stranded configuration and a GC content similar to that calculated for the DNA of infective particles. In the case of KBSH-virus the majority of the DNA had a molecular weight of about 2.7×10^5 daltons consistent with not more than 20 per cent of the nucleic acid of a complete infectious virus. The respective figures obtained for LuIII-virus are 2.3×10^5 daltons and about 15 per cent.

b) Structural Proteins

Data concerning the number and size of the structural proteins are so far only available for LuIII-virus (GAUTSCHI and SIEGL, 1973). Proteins were labelled with radioactive amino acids and infectious virions, incomplete particles, as well as capsids devoid of DNA were extensively purified by repeated banding in CsCl and by sedimentation in sucrose gradients. In contrast to the data reported for other parvoviruses, SDS-polyacrylamide gel electrophoresis provided evidence for the presence of only two structural polypeptides in the infectious virion. A polypeptide with a molecular weight of 62,000 represented 84.5 per cent of the total amount of radioactive amino acids incorporated whereas 15.5 per cent of label was associated with a polypeptide having a molecular weight of 75,000 daltons. Only incomplete or empty particles contained small amounts (about 4 per cent) of an additional third protein with a molecular weight of 69,000 daltons.

Purification of LuIII-virus included incubation of crude viral harvests with receptor destroying enzyme, trypsin, and deoxycholate. It seems possible that such a treatment might have removed the third protein from the infectious virion. Experiments concerned with the synthesis of viral proteins showed, however, that infectious as well as empty particles devoid of the third protein could regularly be isolated from the nucleus of infected cells without prior enzyme digestion (GAUTSCHI et al., 1976). Moreover, a polypeptide with the electrophoretic mobility of the third protein component appears to be synthesized within the nuclei of both infected and uninfected cells at the time virus replication in a synchronized cell culture is at its height. This would suggest the third polypeptide to be a cellular component without any importance for structure, stability, or biologic activity of the virion.

c) Buoyant Density

All tested reference virus strains showed one and the same buoyancy behaviour in CsCl gradients (SIEGL et al., 1971; SIEGL, 1972, 1973). The majority of both infectious and hemagglutinating virions banded at a mean density of 1.39 to 1.41 g/ml and peak amounts of hemagglutinating but noninfectious particles could be detected at densities of 1.305 to 1.32 g/ml. Between these two peaks infectivity titration as well as the hemagglutination test usually revealed a plateau ranging from 1.38 to 1.335 g/ml. On the other hand, determination of the density distribution of ^{3}H-thymidine labelled virus revealed a small peak at 1.44 g/ml, a major fraction consistent with the peak of the infectious virions at 1.39 to 1.41 g/ml, and a further distinct peak located at a medium density of 1.34 to 1.36 g/ml. After isolation and rebanding in CsCl the high density peak as well as the major fraction of infectious virions proved to be homogenous whereas fractions with densities around 1.35 g/ml occasionally yielded small amounts of infectious virions accumulating at 1.4 g/ml. The various particle species have been further characterized with respect to physicochemical and biological properties. It could be shown that particles banding at 1.44 g/ml are infectious, hemagglutinate, and contain a full complement of viral nucleic acid. With exception of their buoyancy they are thus indistinguishable from the majority of complete infectious virions. The denser particle then may be assumed to contain either a lower amount of protein or to have lost a certain quantity of water during some cristallization type of aggregate formation. Unfortunately there are no experimental results favouring any of the two hypotheses.

Upon extraction the hemagglutinating particles accumulating around 1.35 g/ml yielded nucleic acid with a molecular weight of 2.3 to 2.6×10^5 daltons. Such a small piece of DNA represents only 15 to 20 per cent of the nucleic acid of an infectious virion and, in consequence, the term 'incomplete' has been chosen to characterize this particle species. There is strong evidence that the low amount of infectivity usually associated with gradient fractions collected around 1.35 g/ml is due to the presence of some complete infectious virions in aggregates of incomplete particles.

According to electron microscopy, the peak at 1.305 to 1.32, which is exclusively characterized by its high hemagglutination titer, is made up of empty or disrupted capsids.

d) Sedimentation Coefficients

The sedimentation coefficient of KBSH-virus was determined in the preparative ultracentrifuge according to the method suggested by POLSON and VAN REGENMORTEL (1961). Infectious virus recovered from CsCl-gradient fractions with densities of between 1.38 to 1.40 g/ml sedimented with 105 ± 10 Svedberg units and a figure of 72 Svedberg units was calculated for empty capsids isolated from a density of 1.31 g/ml (SIEGL et al., 1971).

The sedimentation behaviour of the various particle species separated by buoyant density centrifugation of LuIII-virus has been analyzed in 5 to 20 per cent sucrose gradients (GAUTSCHI et al., 1974). Infectious virions with a density of 1.41 g/ml sedimented regularly at about 110S. The fraction of incomplete virus banding around 1.35 g/ml, however, obviously represents a still inhomogenous population of particles. Depending on the sample used, figures between 65 to 75S were recorded. Empty capsids (1.31 g/ml), on the other hand, sedimented uniformly with 60S.

e) Resistance to Physical and Chemical Agents

(1) Heat and pH

The reference virus strains KBSH, TVX, and LuIII proved to be as resistant to heating as other parvoviruses. Neither infectivity nor the hemagglutination titer of the viruses in tissue culture medium or glycine buffer pII 9 was affected during incubation at 56° C for 1 hour. The infectivity of density gradient purified fractions of KBSH-virus in 0.15 M veronal acetate buffer pH 7.2, however, was reduced about a hundred-fold when the samples were heated to 75° C for 1 hour (SIEGL et al., 1971).

The decrease of the hemagglutination titers during heating of virus suspensions was proportional to the recorded reduction of infectivity. Moreover, the stability of the hemagglutinin at elevated temperature depended largely on the pH of the suspension medium used (SIEGL et al., 1971). Thus, the hemagglutinating property of the reference virus strains was well preserved between pH 3 and 10 at temperatures of or below 56° C during 1 hour. At higher temperatures, however, the pH had to be adjusted to pH 3 to 7 to assure further resistance of the hemagglutinin. Comparative studies on the stability of H-1, H-3, RV, X-14, MVM, and PPV led to the very same results and are compatible with the observations of GREEN (1965) on the behaviour of H-1 virus.

(2) *Organic Solvents and Na-Deoxycholate*

The viruses are resistant to the action of choloroform, ether, and ethanol. Treatment of tissue culture harvests with choloroform and Freon for 10 to 30 minutes at room temperature in addition offers an extensive means of achieving at least partial purification of virus suspensions. Incubation in the presence of 0.1 to 1.0 per cent Na-deoxycholate for as long as 36 hours neither affected the infectivity nor the hemagglutination titer of the tested virus samples (SIEGL et al., 1971).

(3) *Enzymes*

A broad variety of enzymes such as DNase, RNase, papain, pepsin, and trypsin has been frequently used in the preparation of virus samples. None of these enzymes showed any destructive effect on either the infectivity or the hemagglutinin of complete virus particles even after extending the treatment for as long as 18 hours.

(4) *Storage*

During more than ten years experience with the viruses isolated from permanent human cell lines, storage of virus samples never gave rise to any problems. Lyophilized tissue culture harvests or glycine extracts could be readily stored without any loss in hemagglutinin or infectivity and only insignificant changes were observed when fluid samples were kept at −20° or −70° C for as long as three years. At refrigerator temperature the virus titers of such suspensions remained stable for a mean time of about three weeks.

For storage of highly purified virus suspensions, however, the use of phosphate buffered saline, pH 7.4, should be avoided in favour of Tris buffer pH 7.6 or 0.01 M EDTA pH 7.0 since, in this suspension medium, a moderate but nevertheless significant loss of infectivity occurred after freezing at −20° C (SIEGL et al., 1971).

4. Antigenicity and Serologic Properties

For virus strains KBSH, TVX, and LuIII it was possible to show the presence of a neutralizable, a complement-fixing, as well as a hemagglutinating antigen within the virus particle (HALLAUER et al., 1971, 1972). At the present time there is no evidence concerning the physicochemical characteristics of the

complement-fixing antigen. Density gradient studies, however, led to the conclusion that the hemagglutinin is located on the protein shell of the viruses and,
very likely, is identical with the capsomeres (SIEGL et al., 1971).

a) Characteristics of the Hemagglutinin

The interaction between viral hemagglutinin and susceptible red blood cells
has been investigated by HALLAUER and KRONAUER (1962) and HALLAUER et al.
(1972). According to these studies, the hemagglutinin of all virus strains can be
readily detected by means of guinea pig, human group 0, and rat red blood cells.
These erythrocytes are agglutinated without significant differences in titer at 4°,
room temperature, and at 37° C. Variation of pH between 6.6 and 8.5 had no
effect on HA-titers. Resuspension of agglutinated RBC's in buffer of pH 9.0 at
room temperature, however, resulted in a complete elution of virus within about
30 minutes. Erythrocytes processed in this way reacted again with the hemagglutinin of all virus strains without any reduction in HA-titer as well as with
influenza virus strain PR8.   On the other hand, pretreatment of erythrocytes
with RDE or with various myxovirus strains (e.g. influenza virus type A, B, and
Newcastle disease virus) rendered RBC's inagglutinable to all parvovirus strains
under study. We may assume, therefore, that the cell receptors are the same for
both myxoviruses and parvoviruses, but binding of parvoviruses is neither
paralleled nor followed by any enzymatic degradation of the receptor site.

b) Hemagglutination Pattern

All virus strains isolated from continuous cell lines reacted regularly and
strongly with human, guinea pig, and rat erythrocytes and, to a variable degree,
with RBC's of many other species (HALLAUER et al., 1972). The extent to which
erythrocytes of various species are agglutinated by a certain parvovirus is influenced, however, both by the amount of hemagglutinin and the genetic background of the RBC's included in the test. A reliable comparison of the hemagglutination patterns of all reference strains of the tissue culture contaminants
with those of other parvoviruses, therefore, could be achieved only by using
both hemagglutinins adjusted to a similar HA-titer (1:4096 to 1:8192 for guinea
pig cells) and RBC's of the same batches. The results obtained in this way by
HALLAUER and coworkers (1972) are included in Table 8 (p. 88) and may be
briefly summarized as follows:

All three reference strains as well as H-1, RV, RTV, H-3, X-14, MVM, and
PPV proved to be indistinguishable with respect to their reactivity with human
group 0, guinea pig, and rat erythrocytes. With exception of MVM, all viruses
also readily agglutinated rhesus monkey RBC's.

Clear cut differences in the range of agglutinable cell types, however, were
revealed when additional RBC's of mammalian and avian origin were included
in the test. Only KBSH, TVX, LuIII, PPV, RTV, and H-1 reacted regularly
with fowl and goose erythrocytes. KBSH and PPV, both belonging to the same
serotype, showed a weak agglutination or no agglutination at all with mouse,
rabbit, hamster, sheep, horse, cattle, pig, cat, and dog RBC's.   Finally, the spe-
cificity of MVM proved in so far outstanding as hemagglutination with this virus
was restricted to the use of human, guinea pig, mouse, rat, hamster, and dog cells.

c) Hemadsorption

In contrast to the well documented ability of the parvoviruses to agglutinate RBC's of various species, results concerning the adsorption of such erythrocytes onto the surface of infected tissue culture cells are contradictory (KILHAM and OLIVIER, 1959; PORTELLA, 1964; CARTWRIGHT *et al.*, 1969). Early attempts to detect hemadsorption with the virus strains referred to in this chapter gave negative results (HALLAUER and KRONAUER, 1962). In a more recent study, however, a low degree of adsorption of human red blood cells onto HeLa cells infected with KBSH-virus could be observed (HALLAUER *et al.*, 1972). The reaction is nevertheless without any value for the detection of virus-infected cells since it occurred only at a rather late stage of virus replication when cell-associated virus had reached high HA-titers and cultures already exhibited a clear cut cytopathic effect. Under similar conditions, hemadsorption was completely absent in tissue cultures infected with TVX and LuIII viruses.

d) Serologic Properties

Using reference antisera prepared in rabbits against several of the virus strains recovered from 36 out of 41 permanent human cell lines all isolates could be classified by means of HI-tests in three distinct serologic groups (HALLAUER *et al.*, 1971). The great majority (29) of the isolates, represented by strain KBSH, proved to be closely related to, or even identical, with porcine parvovirus. Hemagglutination of 8 isolates, represented by TVX-virus, was regularly inhibited to a low degree by a high titer anti-H-1 serum, but specific antisera against TVX virus never interfered with the hemagglutination reaction of H-1 virus. Finally, a third serotype is confined to LuIII virus obtained from only one cell strain and showing no serologic relationship to any of the so far known parvoviruses (see also Table 9, p. 90).

Immunofluorescent staining of cell cultures infected with KBSH, TVX, or LuIII virus supported the close serologic relatedness of PPV and KBSH virus as suggested already by HAI-testing (SIEGL *et al.*, 1971). Moreover, this technique proved as inefficient as the HAI-test in disclosing an additional antigen in common for all three reference strains (unpublished observation).

5. Cultural Characteristics

The viruses dealt with in this chapter have all been isolated from various strains of stable cell lines. A description and evaluation of their biological characteristics is therefore subjected to quite another scale than that used during discussion of *in vitro* and *in vivo* features of the other parvoviruses capable of replication without a helper virus. Many different questions such as for example, origin, biological significance, latent behaviour, sudden appearance and disappearance of virus multiplication in apparently normal and uninfected tissue cultures, constitute a rather complex problem, a possible explanation of which, despite of many thorough experimental investigations, cannot be given at the present time without taking refuge in speculation.

a) Parvovirus Contaminated Cell Lines

(1) Origin of Isolates

Since HALLAUER and KRONAUER (1962) detected a particulate hemagglutinin (which subsequently proved to be a parvovirus) as a latent contaminant in certain human cell lines, a total of 43 cell strains from 7 stable cell lines (see Table 6) has been tested for the presence of the agents by means of the alkaline extraction method described by HALLAUER and KRONAUER (1960, 1962, 1965). Thereby, isolation attempts were successful in as many as 38 cases yielding three serologically distinct groups of viruses (HALLAUER et al., 1971).

Table 6. *Origin and Frequency of Isolation of the Parvoviruses Contaminating Permanent Human Cell Lines (According to HALLAUER et al., 1971)*

Cell line	Number of Strains		Antigenic Type of Virus		
	Tested	Infected	KBSH (PPV)	TVX	LuIII
HeLa	18	17	13	4	—
KB	9	9	9	—	—
HEp-2	3	2	2	—	—
Detroit 30A	1	—	—	—	—
FL-Amnion	8	8	5	3	—
Lu 106	3	2	—	1	1
Lu 132	1	—	—	—	—
Total	43	38	29	8	1

The infected cell strains almost exclusively had been obtained from a number of European institutes. It was a common observation that strains, already upon arrival in the laboratory, showed signs of degeneration, and, following extraction with alkaline buffers, delivered a large amount of hemagglutinating virus. Others, on the contrary, were of normal aspect and only yielded virus after 1 to 150 serial passages. The circumstances of isolation, serologic typing of the recovered parvoviruses, determination of host cell range (see section 5 b) as well as screening of sera of human and animal origin for specific antibodies (HALLAUER et al., 1971) provided the possibility of answering, at least partially, some questions concerning the origin of infection:

(i) The observation that different cell strains of one and the same stable cell line harboured viruses belonging to different serologic groups strongly reduces the probability that these permanent cell lines were infected "de origine" with the isolates and then remained in a carrier state up to the passage of discovery.

(ii) The possibility of contamination of freshly obtained cell strains in the course of experimental investigations cannot be denied. However, recovery of similar agents obviously occurred in distant laboratories not dealing with the same or related viruses. The source of contamination, therefore, is wide spread and has to be looked for in the methods and ingredients used during routine cultivation of permanent cell lines.

Laboratory workers handling the tissue cultures very probably cannot be considered a source of the viruses since sera of six individuals engaged in culturing the different virus strains for 1 to 10 years were found to be devoid of any detectable amount of specific HI-antibodies. In addition, screening of more than 500 human sera for HI-antibodies to the isolated viruses gave negative results.

The remaining sources of contamination have to be looked for in the materials of biological origin used in routine cultivation of the permanent cell lines such as sera of different species as well as lactalbumin hydrolysate to supplement growth media and enzymes to disperse the cells for passage. After all, however, only sera and enzymes are treated cautiously enough during preparation to allow preservation of viral infectivity, whereas, according to information from the manufacturer, lactalbumin hydrolysate is autoclaved during the production process.

Calf serum had been used without exception by HALLAUER and coworkers in the cultivation of the tested cell lines and, due to its ready availability, most likely is added also to growth media in other laboratories. There was no real evidence, however, that the isolated viruses were picked up in this way since out of 500 bovine sera collected from cattle stocks in Switzerland only one sample was shown to contain HI-antibodies to KBSH-virus (titer 1:40) and two had insignificant HI-titers (1:20) to TVX.

Stimulated by the observation of URBANO (1969) who isolated poliovirus type 2 from several bottles of a commercial trypsin batch, HALLAUER et al. (1971) then suggested that at least those parvoviruses serologically identical with porcine parvovirus might have been introduced into the tissue cultures by use of trypsin extracted from the pancreas of PPV infected pigs. The direct recovery of PPV from commercial trypsin of hog pancreas origin reported recently (CROGHAN et al., 1973) gave strong support to this assumption. On the other hand, the natural host of viruses related serologically to TVX and LuIII remains unknown.

(2) Cultural Behaviour

The carrier state of cell lines with parvoviruses cannot be easily recognized since the cell monolayers show, in most cases, a quite normal aspect or, at best, a slight degree of cell degeneration similar to that in ageing, noninfected cultures. In addition, the contaminating parvovirus is highly cell-bound so that a spontaneous release of viral hemagglutinin is only observed when the cell-associated virus reaches a high concentration. Under these circumstances the extraction of cell-associated virus with alkaline buffers is the most easy and reliable method to detect parvovirus contamination in cell cultures at every passage level. Using this procedure, the behaviour of cell cultures contaminated by parvoviruses could be analysed in a satisfactory manner (HALLAUER et al., 1971).

Some strains yielded very high titers (32,000—250,000 HAU/0.25 ml) of hemagglutinin already at receipt and exhibited a pronounced CPE causing their loss in the first or the early subsequent passages. The majority of the cell strains, however, were at first sight not suspected to carry parvovirus, but yielded virus after a more or less high number of culture passages either continuously during months and even years, or in alternating cycles of passages during which virus could be either easily or not at all detected.

Although permanent latent infections in long-term passaged cell strains are the rule, there is always the possibility that a sudden and fulminant CPE accompanied by an extraordinary high release of virus finally causes the loss of the cell line. Indeed, there was evidence that both number and frequency of passages may induce such an activation of the carrier state. Additional observations suggested a close relationship existing between stimulation of active virus synthesis and circumstantial factors influencing the physiologic state of the affected cell. Thus, many cell strains yielded hemagglutinin after shipping or mailing whereas others became "positive" directly or a few passages after thawing of cell samples stored at $-70°$ C.

b) Experimentally Infected Cell Cultures

(1) Host Cell Range

In analogy with other parvoviruses, the susceptibility of various cell systems for virus strains KBSH, TVX, and LuIII has been investigated (HALLAUER et al., 1972). Cell lines known to harbour frequently parvoviruses were only tested following a rigorous examination demonstrating their freedom from any contamination. The results thus obtained are included in Tables 10 and 11 (pp. 92, 93).

The three reference virus strains multiplied in all human cell lines tested. In contrast to H-1, H-3, RV, and MVM, however, they could never be propagated successfully in any cell line of rodent (mouse, rat, and hamster) origin. Virus strain KBSH was in so far exceptional as this virus could be readily cultivated in the continuous pig kidney cell line PK 15 and, in addition, was supposed to multiply in a strain of embryonic calf kidney cells as well as in a "transformed" strain of cat kidney fibroblasts. HALLAUER and coworkers (1972) concluded that the observed cultural behaviour of KBSH virus is consistent with the close serologic relationship existing between KBSH and porcine parvovirus.

The high susceptibility of established cell lines for KBSH, TVX, and LuIII-virus had no counter part in attempts to cultivate the viruses in primary or secondary cultures of human embryonic fibroblasts or human amnion cells. Though presence of viral hemagglutinin could be demonstrated in these cultures following infection with high input doses for up to 45 days, and occasionally, also in subcultures, progressive multiplication was never observed. Likewise, primary or secondary monolayers of rhesus or patas monkey kidney as well as embryonic fibroblasts of hamster, guinea pig, and chicken origin proved to be not suited for propagation of strains KBSH and TVX.

(2) Virus Multiplication and Cytopathogenicity

The experimental data reported by HALLAUER et al. (1971, 1972,) SIEGL et al. (1972) as well as by SIEGL and GAUTSCHI (1973) and summarized in the following sections, lent support to the assumption that the multiplication of parvovirus KBSH, TVX, and LuIII is strictly governed by cellular helper functions occurring only briefly during the replication cycle of a susceptible cell. In consequence, the degree of virus multiplication as well as the development of CPE in a certain culture system depend both on the virus dose inoculated and, mainly, on the growth activity of the cells. It is then easy to understand why best results in the propagation of the viruses were obtained if infection of the cultures took place either at the time of cell seeding or at a stage when the cell monolayers had reached only about 50 per cent confluence. Moreover, low level infections in completely confluent cell sheets could be readily activated by subculturing the infected monolayers at a low cell density (HALLAUER and KRONAUER, 1962; HALLAUER et al., 1972).

The beginning of CPE usually was signalled by diffuse granulation. Subsequent rounding up of cells then resulted in roughening of the cell sheet and, following detachment of single or groups of pyknotic cells, complete destruction of the monolayer could be observed. Such a type of CPE was found to be characteristic for all reference virus strains and susceptible tissue cultures tested (HALLAUER et al., 1971). It only developed, however, when cultures having a high mitotic index were inoculated. Otherwise local detachment of rounded cells only led to mere thinning of the affected cell sheet.

Immunofluorescent staining of KBSH- as well as of LuIII-virus infected tissue cultures revealed virus-specific antigen both in the cytoplasm and in the nucleus of infected cells (SIEGL et al., 1972; SIEGL and GAUTSCHI, 1973). Whereas intracytoplasmic fluorescence was observed in 90 to 100 per cent of a tissue culture's cells within a few hours following infection with an appropriate virus dose (5 to 10 m.o.i.), the number of cells showing intranuclear viral antigen 6 to 10 hours p.i. closely reflected the percentage of cells undergoing mitosis. Appearance of intranuclear antigen started with the distribution of fluorescing granules throughout the nucleoplasm. Subsequently, these granules grew and occasionally condensed into large masses until nothing but the areas occupied by the nucleoli appeared unstained. Upon retraction from the nuclear membrane the granular masses behaved like an undifferentiated inclusion body. Such inclusion bodies frequently were present in the nuclei of paired cells. At later stages of viral replication, accumulation of intranuclear fluorescence was found associated with spread of viral antigen back into the cytoplasm. Finally, heavy staining pyknotic nuclei were lost from the shell sheet.

Both histologic and ultrahistologic studies of KBSH-virus infected KB-cells (SIEGL et al., 1972) yielded results fitting well into the above picture. By means of H & E staining intranuclear morphologic alterations could be observed as early as 14 hours after infection. These cytopathologic changes consisted either in an accumulation of eosinophilic to basophilic granulation between the nucleoli and the marginated nuclear chromatine or in the appearance of typical basophilic inclusion bodies. Even under optimal cultural conditions, i.e. after infection of cell cultures of outstanding high mitotic activity (mitotic index about 6 per cent) with maximum infectivity doses, basophilic inclusions were present in not more than 4 to 6 per cent of all infected cells.

First ultrahistological evidence for virus synthesis within the nuclei of infected cells consisted in the demonstration of groups of either empty virus particles or of particles containing a prominent heavy staining core about 15 mμ in size in the nucleoplasm. The onset of intranuclear virus replication and, concurrently, the beginning of pathologic cellular response was signalled by the arrangement of virus particles at the border of nuclear chromatin and the depletion of the interchromatin areas. As a final step the affected nuclei showed severe signs of vacuolization frequently associated with splitting of the nuclear membrane.

(3) *Virus Synthesis*

Based on the obvious correlation between viral replication and the mitotic index of the infected cell sheet (HALLAUER *et al.*, 1972; SIEGL *et al.*, 1972), SIEGL and GAUTSCHI (1973) attempted to study the synthesis of parvovirus LuIII in synchronously growing cells. For this purpose either monolayer or spinner cultures of HeLa cells were synchronized for DNA synthesis. Cells thus accumulating in late G-1 or early S-phase of the cell cycle were then infected at various times following release from the synchronization block.

Immunofluorescent staining of infected cultures showed that early events in the multiplication of LuIII virus, *i.e.* adsorption, and penetration of viral antigen into the cytoplasm, were not controlled by cellular physiology. Maximum numbers of cells showing intracytoplasmic fluorescence were present about 2 to 3 hours p.i. whether randomly growing or synchronized cultures had been infected. As indicated by the results of experiments using radiolabelled virus, more then 95 per cent of the inoculum adsorbed to the cells within only 20 minutes at 4° C and, following warming of the cultures to 37° C, viral nucleic acid was transported to the nuclei within 60 to 120 minutes (SIEGL and GAUTSCHI, 1975).

Early studies suggested the appearance of intracytoplasmic fluorescence to be indicative for a first transcription and translation during virus synthesis (SIEGL *et al.*, 1972; SIEGL and GAUTSCHI, 1973 a, b). More recent investigations, however, led to the conclusion that development of intracytoplasmic fluorescence reflects nothing but the uptake of an excess of viral antigens by the infected cells (SIEGL, GAUTSCHI, and TRACHSEL, unpublished).

Following the transport of viral nucleic acid into the nuclei, further events in the replication of LuIII-virus were found to be limited by the availability of cellular helper functions. Whether infected at the beginning of S-phase or 3 to 4 hours later at the height of cellular DNA synthesis, intranuclear viral antigen was detected as early as 10 hours after release of cells from the synchronization block. Intranuclear fluorescence then increased linearly between 10 and 16 hours. Synthesis of cell-associated infective and hemagglutinating virus was first detected between 8 and 10 hours and, like incorporation of ^{3}H-thymidine into progeny viral DNA, strictly paralleled the accumulation of intranuclear viral antigen (SIEGL and GAUTSCHI, 1973 a, b). Since viral adsorption, penetration, and transport of viral nucleic acid into the nucleus takes about 3 hours, the status of "physiologic competence" necessary for successful completion of virus multiplication has been assumed to be identical with events in late S-phase of the cell cycle.

Detailed studies concerning the synthesis of both viral DNA and proteins lent further support to the above conclusions (SIEGL and GAUTSCHI, 1976; GAUTSCHI *et al.*, 1976). Between 9 and 10 hours after infection in early S-phase the selective extraction of low molecular weight DNA and sedimentation analysis revealed the beginning synthesis of a double-stranded, replicative viral DNA (dsDNA) sedimenting with 14 to 16 S and banding at 1.715 g/ml in CsCl. With progressing time the sedimentation spectrum developed a small additional peak at 24 S and a broad shoulder between 18 and 22 S. According to the results obtained by electron microscopy, the dsDNA molecules were comparable in length to the single-stranded molecules of progeny viral DNA a small number of which contributed to the 24 S peak. Molecules of similar length but showing a varying amount of single-stranded branches were isolated from fractions with sedimentation constants between 18 and 22 S. This DNA species was assumed to represent a replicative intermediate form (RIF) in the synthesis of progeny viral DNA.

A not completely understood finding concerned the appearance of double-stranded DNA molecules about three times as long as viral dsDNA within the 24 S peak. Some of these molecules were reported to contain two short side chains located at a distance comparable with the length of viral DNA. This observation and the possibility to dissociate at least part of the large molecules at alkaline pH into subunits sedimenting with the characteristics of single-stranded viral DNA gave rise to the assumption that the double-stranded DNA at 24 S represents nothing but aggregated viral dsDNA. On the other hand, however, denaturation yielded in addition single-stranded molecules with about three times the molecular weight of dsDNA.

The appearance of a double-stranded replicative viral DNA concomitantly with the first detectable synthesis of progeny viral nucleic acid and shortly after the cells reached the status of "physiologic competence" rised the question whether the "factors" provided by the cell's metabolism are responsible for the formation of dsDNA or for the synthesis of progeny viral DNA only. Attempts to follow the formation of dsDNA by infection of synchronized cell cultures with ³H-thymidine labelled LuIII-virus and by analysing the buoyancy behaviour of extracted labelled DNA molecules were only partially conclusive (SIEGL and GAUTSCHI, 1976). Labelled DNA molecules were recovered up to 3.5 hours following infection in early S-phase of the cell cycle and a clear cut peak of radioactivity with a density of dsDNA developed as early as 4.5 hours p.i. already in mid S-phase. Since, however, less than 10 per cent of the total radioactive DNA inoculated could be recovered by the extraction procedure applied and the cell cultures were synchronized only to a degree of about 70 per cent, the formation of dsDNA might have indicated only synthetic events in that fraction of the cells which escaped synchronization.

GAUTSCHI et al. (1976) have analysed the synthesis of proteins in LuIII infected HeLa cells. Nuclei of cells infected in early S-phase were isolated at various times during the cell cycle and nuclear proteins were separated into a salt soluble fraction, histones, and nonhistone chromosomal proteins. The experimental results suggested that virus replication did not interfere with the synthesis of soluble nuclear proteins up to 10 hours p.i. At later times, however, incorporation of label into the soluble fraction of infected nuclei increased significantly. About the same proved true for the synthesis of nonhistone chromosomal proteins. Differences in the incorporation of labelled amino acids in infected and mock-infected cells again became evident only about 10 hours after infection. Moreover, lacking differences between the values recorded for synthesis of histones in mock-infected and in virus-infected cells suggested that infection with LuIII virus did not disturb the synthetic events in cellular S-phase.

According to electrophoresis on polyacrylamide gels, the histone proteins extracted at different times after infection proved free of any of the polypeptides characteristic for the purified mature virus particle. For the first time these polypeptides could be demonstrated in a significant amount in extracts of nonhistone chromosomal proteins 11 to 12 hours post infection. Labelling with tritiated leucine and valine revealed both the two main species of viral polypeptides and an additional polypeptide migrating like the third "viral" polypeptide present in incomplete particles. Yet, at the same time, such a protein was synthesized in a significant amount in mock-infected cells.

Eleven to 12 hours p.i. the two specific viral polypeptides were present in the fraction of soluble nuclear proteins only at a very low concentration. With progressing time, however, their amount increased drastically. Since accumulation of viral proteins could be correlated with the accumulation of infectious, mature virions as well as with empty viral capsids, the appearance of the two viral polypeptides within the fraction of soluble nuclear proteins was assumed to be indicative for the maturation of LuIII-virus. Replication of viral DNA, on the other hand, was thought to take place in close association with cellular non-histone chromosomal proteins.

6. Pathogenicity

HALLAUER and KRONAUER (1962) reported that the first isolates of the hemagglutinating tissue culture contaminants did not multiply in the embryonated hen's egg even after different modes of infection. In addition, no indication for any pathogenic action could be recorded when adult albino mice were inoculated intracerebrally or when newborn mice were inoculated either by the intracerebral or intraperitoneal route. When the studies were extended to syrian hamsters, both adult and neonatal animals of this species also proved to be insusceptible to TVX. Some further preliminary results suggested that KBSH-virus is neither pathogenic for adult mice and hamsters nor for newborn mice. Baby hamsters injected intraperitoneally with 10^4 $TCID_{50}/0.03$ ml of the virus within 24 hours after birth, however, developed HI-antibody titers of 1:80 at 6 month of age (HALLAUER et al., 1972).

More detailed studies have been done with LuIII-virus. SOIKE and coworkers (1976) were able to adapt and to passage this virus in newborn hamsters. Already in the second passage some of the animals inoculated intraperitoneally or subcutaneously with a tissue homogenate (lung, liver, spleen, and kidney) died within four days and at passage level four all animals inoculated either by the intraperitoneal, the intracerebral, or the oral route succumbed between four to six days p.i.

At necropsy, principal pathology consisted in an extensive intestinal hemorrhage, hepatitis, petechial hemorrhages in the kidney, and a paleness of the lung suggesting some anemia. Concomitantly with this finding, virus was readily recovered from the intestine and, in decreasing amounts, from kidneys, liver, heart, spleen, lung, and brain of the animals.

Besides that, LuIII-virus was shown to cross the placenta of pregnant hamsters. When the animals were infected with 10^3 newborn hamster DL_{50} of virus at 2, 4, 6, 8, 10, and 12 days of gestation, transplacental infection could be demonstrated following inoculation at days 8, 10, and 12 with a frequency of abortions of 77, 44, and 19 per cent, respectively. Virus was recovered from all fetuses, placentas, and abortuses at 8 and 10 days and from 1 of 6 animals inoculated at day 12. Interestingly, however, attempts to isolate the virus from maternal lung, liver, spleen, kidney, or heart were negative.

IV. General Survey

For years, a study concerning the characteristics of parvoviruses appeared to describe a mere laboratory problem. With one exception—the causative agent included in feline panleukopenia, feline ataxia, and mink enteritis—potential members of the genus, whether isolated from human, rat, hamster, mouse, pig, calf, or dog tissue specimens, were encountered by chance and, due to their unknown role as pathogens, only enlarged the group of "viruses in search of disease". Nevertheless, the first data obtained during early investigations clearly indicated that, with the discovery of parvoviruses, an important gap then still present in the DNA-virus class could be filled.

The morphological and physicochemical characteristics (see Table 7) of the agents as a whole are unique among those of all other known animal and plant viruses. Only bacteriophage $\Phi X\,174$ (SINSHEIMER, 1959) was found to share a complex of similar properties but the characteristics of the parvoviruses and of $\Phi X\,174$ are nevertheless not congruent. The virions of both phage and animal viruses are isometric, nonenveloped particles about 18 to 26 nm in diameter. They contain a single-stranded DNA with molecular weight of between 1.5 to 2.2×10^6 daltons. Whereas, however, the DNA of $\Phi X\,174$ is a circular molecule, only linear single strands have been recovered so far from parvoviruses.

A further difference may consist in both number and arrangement of the protein subunits within the capsid. The protein shell of $\Phi X\,174$ is known to be composed of only 12 distinct and relatively large capsomeres located at the vertices of an icosahedron (TROMANS and HORNE, 1961). On the other hand, analysis of the fine structure of several parvoviruses suggested that, in this case, the more stable but similar sized capsid is constructed of 32 subunits. Despite this repeated observation, composition and symmetry of the capsid is still a matter of discussion. The most recent model has been proposed by KONGSVIK and coworkers (1974) who, on the basis of the relative amount of viral polypeptides within a H-1 virus particle, reconsidered the possibility of an icosahedron made up of only 12 pentamers.

All members of the genus parvovirus are characterized by the ability to agglutinate erythrocytes (see Table 8). As a rule, hemagglutination can be easily demonstrated with guinea pig RBC's and most of the viruses agglutinate additional cells from a broad variety of species. In the case of feline panleukopenia/mink enteritis virus as well as of the minute virus of canines, however, agglutination is obviously restricted to only one single type of red blood cells, i.e. to those of pig and rhesus monkey origin, respectively. Finally, there is substantial evidence that comparative hemagglutination tests conducted under strictly controlled conditions can be used to distinguish between viruses showing a very close serologic relationship, such as, for example, H-1 and HT-virus.

Parvoviruses were found to be serologically unrelated to other DNA viruses and, in addition, share no common group antigen. Comparative cross hemagglutination inhibition as well as neutralization tests revealed that the various isolates may belong to at least 9 serologically distinct subgroups represented by the prototype viruses RV, H-1, RTV, PPV, TVX, LuIII, FPV, MVM, and bovine parvovirus (HADEN) (see Table 9). The antigenic structure of HB-virus isolated

Table 7. *Physicochemical Characteristics of Parvovirus Reference Strains*

Virus	Virion				ss DNA		Stability			References
	Size (nm)	Mol. wt. ($\times 10^6$)	Density in CsCl (g/ml)	Sed. coefficient	% per particle	Mol. wt. ($\times 10^6$)	Ether	65°/30 min	pH 3	
RV	18—28	6.6	1.38—1.47	110	25.7	1.2—1.7	+	+	+	113, 131, 162, 174, 210, 215
RTV	19—21	5.7	1.41	110	27.2	1.6	+	+	+	232, *
H-1	20—30	6.6	1.39	110	25.7	1.7—2.3	+	+	+	75, 76, 77, 113, 174, 257, 268
MVM	19—28		1.41—1.43	110		1.2—2.0	+	+	+	42, 43, 174
PPV	20—28	5.3	1.37—1.39	105	26.5	1.4	++	++	++	28, 171,
KBSH	19—22		1.39							226, 232
BPV (HADEN)	23—28						+	+	+	1, 5, 236
FPV/MEV	21—24	5.9	1.41		28.5	1.7	+	+	+	106, 108, 242
MVC	18—20		1.41				+	+	+	18
Lu III	19—22	5.7	1.41	110	28.0	1.6	+	+	+	227, 232
TVX	19—22		1.39				+	+	+	232

* Siegl and coworkers, unpublished

Table 8. *Hemagglutination*

Viruses isolated from:		Range of								
		Human	Monkey	Guinea pig	Rat	Hamster	Mouse	Gerbil	Rabbit	Agouti
I. Rat	RV	+++a +++	+++ ++	+++ +++	++ +++	++ ++	+++ ++	–	– –	+++
	H-3	++ +++	+++ ++	+++ +++	+++ +++	++ +++	++ ++	–	++ (+)	+++
	X-14	++	++	+++	+++	++	++		(+)	
	RTV	+++	+++	+++	+++	+++	++		–	
II. Human (or rat?)	H-1	++ +++	++ ++	+++ +++	++ +++	+++ ++	++ ++	+	– –	+++
	HT	–	–	+++	–	+++	–	–	–	+++
	HB	–	–	+++	++	++	++	–	–	–
III. Mouse	MVM	++	–	+++	++	++	++		–	
IV. Pig	PPV	+++	++	+++	+++	(+)	+		–	
*V. Bovines*b	HADEN	+		+	+	+	–		–	
*VI. Felines & Mink*b FPV/MEV				–			–			
*VII. Canines*b	MVC	–	+	–						
VIII. Human cell lines	KBSH	+++	+++	+++	+++	(+)	+		–	
	TVX	+++	+++	+++	+++	(+)	+		–	
	LuIII	+++	++	+++	+++	+++	+++		–	

a The HA-titers were expressed by virus dilutions giving a complete (256) or 50 per cent (82) hemagglutination:

+++ [1:640—1280 (256), 1:1024—8192 (82)],

++   [1:160—320 (256), 1:128—512 (82)],

+   [1:20—80 (256), 1:16—64 (82)],

(+) [1:10 (256), 1:2—8 (82)],

–   [1:10 (256), no reaction (82)].

b No indication of titer is given.

Spectrum of Parvoviruses

susceptible Erythrocytes											References
Sheep	Goat	Horse	Cattle	Pig	Cat	Dog	Chicken	Goose	Duck	Frog	
–		+++			(+)	++	–	–	++		256
+		+	–	(+)	+	+	(+)	–			82
–		+++			++	+	–	–	+++		256
+		++	–	++	++	+++	(+)	+		+	82
+		++	–	+	+	+	(+)	–		–	82
+		++	–	++	++	+++	+	++			82
–		++			++	++	–	++	++		256
+		+	–	+++	++	+++	+	++		++	82
–		–			(+)	–	–	–	+		256
–		–			–	–	–	–	+		256
–		–	–	–		++	(+)	(+)			82
(+)		–	–	–	+	(+)	++	+			82
+	+	+	–		–	+	–	+	+		1, 5, 12, 94, 239
–		–	–	+	–		–				106
–			–	–		–		–			18
(+)		–	–	–	(+)	(+)	++	++		–	82
++		++	(+)	+++	++	+++	++	++		–	82
+		+++	(+)	+	++	+++	++	++			82

The results obtained by TOOLAN (256) and HALLAUER *et al.* (82) are comparable, since both authors tried to standardize the hemagglutination reaction by testing viruses of a similar IIA-titer (1:1280 and 1:4096—8192, respectively) and by using constantly the same batches of erythrocytes in their experiments

Table 9. *Serologic Relationship between Parvoviruses as Revealed by Hemagglutination-Inhibition*

Antisera to	Parvovirus strains														
	"Hamster-osteolytic" viruses							Murine	Feline	Bovine	Canine	Porcine	Isolates from cell cultures		
	RV	H-3	X-14	RTV	H-1	HT	HB	MVM	FPV/MEV	HADEN	MVC	PPV	KBSH	LuIII	TVX
RV	160	80	80	—	—	—	—	—	—	—	—	—	—	—	—
H-3	640	1280	1280	—	—	—	—	—	—	—	—	—	—	—	80
X-14	80	160	160	—	—	—	—	—	—	—	—	—	—	—	—
RTV	—	—	—	2560	—	—	—	—	—	—	—	—	—	80	—
H-1	—	—	—	—	20,480	+	—	—	—	—	—	—	—	—	320
HT	—	—	—	—	+	+	—	—	—	—	—	—	—	—	—
HB	—	—	—	—	—	—	+	—	—	—	—	—	—	—	—
MVM	—	—	—	—	—	—	—	10,240	—	—	—	—	—	—	—
FPV/MEV	—	—	—	—	—	—	—	—	2560	—	—	—	—	—	—
HADEN	—	—	—	—	—	—	—	—	—	256	—	—	—	—	—
MVC	—	—	—	—	—	—	—	—	—	—	2560	—	—	—	—
PPV	—	—	—	—	—	—	—	—	—	—	—	1280	320	—	—
KBSH	—	—	—	—	—	—	—	—	—	—	—	1280	1280	—	—
LuIII	—	—	—	—	—	—	—	—	—	—	—	—	—	2560	—
TVX	—	—	—	—	—	—	—	—	—	—	—	—	—	—	1280

According to HALLAUER et al. (1971), supplemented with data reported by TOOLAN (1964) (HT, HB), JOHNSON et al. (1967) (FPV), BACHMANN (1971) and STORZ et al. (1972) (HADEN), BINN et al. (1970) (MVC), and SIEGL et al. (unpublished) (FPV, HB, MVM) by TOOLAN (1964) as well as the minute virus of canines (MVC) has not been clarified completely. According to very recent hemagglutination inhibition tests which included the listed prototype strains with the exception of bovine parvovirus, however, both HB and MVC are of distinct antigenicity (SIEGL and coworkers, unpublished).

Besides the structural properties and the outstanding resistance of parvoviruses as evident from their ability to withstand heating to 70° C, the whole group is especially characterized by an exceptional relationship between virus multiplication and the mitotic activity of susceptible host cells. It has been postulated that this close association between virus synthesis and an activated cellular physiologic state reflects a partial inability of the viruses to code for their replication. To a certain extent the reliability of such a conclusion can be judged on the basis of rough calculations repeatedly made up during early studies concerned with the protein constituents of the virions. The informational content of viral DNA was found to suffice only for the two main viral polypeptides whereas coding for the additional third polypeptide would exceed the informational capacity of the nucleic acid.

Some characteristics of the cellular helper functions required for viral replication have been derived from studies based on the multiplication of RV, H-1, LuIII, and MVM in synchronously growing cell cultures. Though adsorption, penetration, and uncoating of the tested viruses obviously occurred at all stages of the cell cycle, synthesis of infective and hemagglutinating progeny virus only started after most, if not all, of the DNA genom of an infected cell had been duplicated. More detailed analysis then suggested that cellular physiologic competence in late S- or early G-2 phase is equivalent to initiation of the synthesis of a double-stranded viral DNA replicative form upon which synthesis of both progeny viral DNA and viral hemagglutinin is dependent (RHODE, 1974a, b; SIEGL and GAUTSCHI, 1976; GAUTSCHI et al., 1976). Since, in addition, replication of viral DNA obviously is confined to the nuclear chromatin, the required helper functions might be identical with those normal cellular processes governing duplication of chromatin late in S-phase.

The strict control of parvovirus multiplication by certain functions displayed only shortly during the division cycle of a susceptible cell provides the basis for the pathogenicity of these viruses. Regardless of whether the data were obtained from experimental animal studies or from the few known cases where a parvovirus plays a role as an etiologic agent of a particular disease, they all suggest the final clinico-pathologic spectrum of alterations to result directly from the involvement of rapidly growing tissues. Thus, infection of pregnant animals led to an accumulation of parvoviruses within the placenta and the fetuses whereas the tissues of the mother largely remained unaffected. The outcome of infection varied with the state of development of the embryo at the time infection occurred and consisted in resorption of the embryo, abortions, or malformations. In experiments with newborn rodents the developing skeleton represents the main target of viral attack and the classic syndrome of feline ataxia could be traced back to a specific destruction of the neonatal cerebellar outer germinal layer by feline panleukopenia virus. Finally, the reduced but nevertheless potential pathogenicity of parvoviruses for an adult organism is again correlated with

Table 10. *Host-Cell Range of Parvoviruses in Primary Cell Cultures*

Cell cultures	Parvovirus strains								
	RV	H-1	MVM	PPV	FPV	HADEN	MVC	KBSH	TVX
Rat, embryonic	+	+	+				—	—	—
Hamster, embryonic	+	+							
Hamster kidney	—	—							
Mouse, embryonic			+	—			—		
Mouse kidney			+						
Guinea pig kidney							—	—	—
Rabbit kidney						—	—		
Pig, kidney and testicle	—			+	—		—		
Bovine, embryonic lung, kidney, testicle				—	—	+ +			
Feline, kidney, lung					— —	—	—		
Mink cells					+				
Ferret cells					+				
Dog cells					+				
Monkey cells				—	—	—	—		
Rhesus kidney				—	—		—	—	—
Human, embryonic	—	—					—	—	—
Human amnion	—	—						—	—
Chicken, embryonic	—	—		—	—	—		—	—
References	131, 150, 180, 190, 260, 257	15, 180, 190, 260, 257	42, 195	4, 27, 28, 171	20, 97, 101	1, 11, 94, 95, 239, 271	18	82	82

Table 11. Host-Cell Range of Parvoviruses in Permanent Cell Lines

Cell lines		Parvovirus strains											References
Species	Strain	RV	RTV	MVM	H-1	PPV	HADEN	FPV/MEV	MVC	KBSH	TVX	LuIII	
Rat	AT	+	+	+	+						−	−	15, 82
	Nephroma	+	+	+	+								209
Hamster	BHK-21	+	−	+	+	−		−		−	−		15, 17, 82
	BHK-35	+	−	+	+	−		−		−	−		82
	HaK			+	−	−				−	−		260
Mouse	L	−	−	+	−	−				−			82
	L 929	−	−	+	−								154
Human	HeLa	−	−	−	+	+	−	−		+	+	+	82, 260
	HeLa-S₃	−	−	−	+	+				+	+	+	260
	KB	−	−	−	+	+		−	−	+	+	+	17, 82
	HEp-2	−	−	−	+	+		−	−	+	+	+	17, 82, 260
	Lu 106	−	−	−	+	+		−	−	+	+	+	17, 82
	Lu 132	−	−	−	+	+		−					82
	FL (amnion)				+								17, 82, 260
	AV₃ (amnion)												154
	Liver (Chang)				+								260
	Intestine (Henle)				+								260
	Conjunctiva (Chang)				+								260
	NB Shein & Enders				+	+							141
	Heart (Salk)				+								260
Monkey	LLC-MK₂			−	−				−	−	−	−	17, 260
	Rita									−	−		82
	Vero	−	−	−	+	−			−	−	−	−	82
	Chimpanzee Liver				+	+							260
Pig	PK 15	−	−	+	+	+				+	−	−	82
Cattle	MDBK									+			17, 82
Cat	NLFK							+	−				108
Dog	MDCK												82
	WRCC								+		−		17
Rabbit	RK 13	−	−	−	−	−				−	−		17, 82
	SIRC	−	−	−	−	−				−	−		82

the availability of replicating cells. In the case of feline panleukopenia/mink enteritis, the destructive action of the virus proved mainly associated with cellular differentiation in the lymphopoietic and erythropoietic organs as well as with the constantly proliferating tissues of the intestines.

There is still a final problem linked to the pathogenic mechanism of parvovirus infections. These agents behave in general as latent viruses. Their persistence in an infected organism is usually paralleled by the presence of large amounts of circulating antibodies. Derangement of the equilibrium between virus multiplication and the state of specific immunity by drugs or other therapeutic treatment with immunosuppressive effect may result in an activation and manifestation of parvovirus infections in regenerating tissues. An instructive example for the possible consequences has been reported by ENGLER *et al.* (1966), who noticed a marked delay in the healing process of osseous wounds in H-1 infected hamsters.

Despite the repeatedly reported isolation of several of the described parvoviruses from tissue specimens of human origin, there is at present no really convincing evidence that one of the viruses might be involved in human disease. However, the application of immune electron microscopy in the search of the causative agents of acute infectious nonbacterial gastroenteritis and of human hepatitis A recently has led to the discovery of parvovirus-like particles in filtrates of feces collected during acute illness (KAPIKIAN *et al.*, 1972, 1973; FEINSTONE *et al.*, 1974). The characteristically envelopeless and isometric particles were 27 nm in diameter. They banded in CsCl gradients at densities around 1.4 g/ml. The so-called "Norwalk agent" of acute nonbacterial gastroenteritis proved serologically unrelated to the hepatitis A candidate virus and particles of the latter virus did not aggregate in the presence of anti RV antibodies.

Detailed characterization of both "Norwalk" and the hepatitis A candidate agent was so far hampered by the fact that, despite extensive attempts in various laboratories, none of the isolates could be cultivated *in vitro*. In studies with human volunteers, however, feeding of filtrates containing either virus resulted in the development of the respective clinical symptoms as well as in the appearance of specific antibodies. Successful propagation of the agents and induction of disease in an animal model system only has been reported for hepatitis A. MAYNARD and colleagues (1974), inoculating either a human stool filtrate rich in the 27 nm particles or particles purified by banding in CsCl gradients, were able to induce viral hepatitis in chimpanzees and marmosets, respectively. This observation is in line with the experimental results of DEINHARDT *et al.* (1967) and of PROVOST *et al.* (1973) suggesting marmoset monkeys to be at present the most convenient model for the study of human hepatitis A.

If the causative agent of human hepatitis A really is a parvovirus and, like other members of this virus group, contains a rather limited genetic information, growing knowledge on the cellular helper functions implicated in parvovirus replication should accelerate the development of a potent *in vitro* culture system. On the same theoretical background, however, one is tempted to speculate whether acute viral hepatitis in adult individuals is nothing but a consequence of massive virus replication in fast proliferating tissues outside the liver or, whether infection will cumulate in clinical disease only in those individuals providing a large amount of dividing cells in an injured, yet, regenerating liver.

V. Addendum

After this review went in press, additional data on several parvoviruses have been published. Thus, the Study Group on *Parvoviridae* of the International Committee on Taxonomy of Viruses presented a summary of the main characteristics of members of the family parvoviridae (BACHMANN *et al.*, 1975). This paper, however, does not include some recent information on the virion of the minute virus of mice (MVM). BOURGIGNON *et al.* (1975) have shown that 99 per cent of complete MVM virions contain only one type of a single-stranded DNA (1.55×10^6 daltons) whereas the remaining 1 per cent of the particles yield a ssDNA of complementary base sequence. Moreover, digestion of viral DNA with the single-strand-specific nuclease S1 and Exo1 suggested 2 to 5 per cent (100—250 nucleotides) of the viral genome to form a double-stranded stable hair-pin structure at the 5'-terminus of the molecule.

CLINTON and HAYASHI (1975) provided evidence for an additional, rather dense (1.47 g/ml) particle in harvests of MVM infected cells. These infective particles contained the same ssDNA molecule as the majority of complete virions (1.42 g/ml); however, differences were noticed with respect to their structural proteins. The dense particles as well as empty viral capsids contained a major polypeptide component with a molecular weight of 72,000 daltons and, as did the complete infectious particles, yielded a second polypeptide of 92,000 daltons. In complete virions, on the other hand, the major component showed a molecular weight of 69,000 daltons. It was assumed that the latter polypeptide is derived from the polypeptide of 72,000 daltons by cleavage in the course of maturation of the virion. Similar results have been obtained by TATTERSALL *et al.* (1975) who estimated the molecular weight of polypeptides in complete virions and empty capsids of MVM to be 82,000, 64,000, and 61,500 daltons. On the basis of peptide maps, combined with sequential harvesting from cells infected under one cycle growth conditions, the authors again concluded that the polypeptide with a molecular weight of 61,500 daltons is a cleavage product of the 64,000 daltons component. The most important observation of this study consisted in the finding that all of the tyrosyl peptides generated during digestion of the 64,000 daltons polypeptide by trypsin or chymotrypsin also occurred in the two other polypeptides.

As regards the replication of parvoviruses, PARRIS *et al.* (1974, 1975) have studied the multiplication of bovine parvovirus (BPV) in cells synchronized for DNA synthesis. Viral infection did not interfere with cellular DNA, RNA, and protein synthesis during S-phase. Subsequently, however, the rate of total RNA and protein synthesis in infected cells decreased significantly whereas, in parallel with the appearance of progeny virus, synthesis of DNA of low molecular weight increased drastically. The morphogenesis of BPV has also been examined at the ultrastructural level in randomly growing bovine fetal lung cell cultures (BATES *et al.*, 1974).

SINGER and TOOLAN (1975) have presented a detailed ultrastructural study of the cytopathology produced by H-1 virus in parasynchronous cultures. At early stages of H-1 virus replication (12 hours p.i.), major ultrastructural changes were confined to the nucleoli. They consisted in a fragmentation and loss of nucleolar fibrous components as well as in an accumulation of "empty" viral particles on the remaining chromatin-like fibers. Eighteen to 36 hours p.i. most virus was located on extranucleolar chromatin fibers and, finally, was liberated concomitantly with progressing cellular degeneration. Interestingly, liberated virions formed extensive paracristalline arrays composed almost exclusively of either complete or empty particles.

In respect to the *in vivo* behaviour of parvoviruses, KILHAM and MARGOLIS (1974) reported that rats infected with RV on the second day of lactation shed the virus in substantial amounts (up to 10^4 $TCID_{50}/0.1$ ml) in the milk. Since infectious virus in addition could be isolated from whole blood and from mamary glands, proliferation of RV in mamary tissue and excretion of virus brought to the gland by the blood stream were postulated to be the chief mechanisms in virolactia. An other member of the "hamster osteolytic" viruses, H-1 virus, was found to induce hepatitis in adult hamsters (HENRY and DIARIO, 1975). Induction of hepatitis was indicated by an increase of serum SGOT and SGPT-values 3 to 9 weeks following inoculation. Diseased livers showed a focal degeneration of hepatic cells. Other symptoms, however, were not evident.

For a long time porcine parvovirus (PPV) has been already assumed to play an important role in pig reproductive failure and fetal malformations. Recently, MENGELING (1975) reported on the naturally occurring transplacental infection with PPV. The virus could be isolated from primary cultures of fetal porcine kidney cells prepared from 3 out of approximately 98 litters collected in an abattoir. Moreover, the presence of high titers of hemagglutination inhibiting (HI) antibody in serum of 0-day-old hysterectomy derived, colostrum-deprived pigs of 3 of 82 litters also indicated transplacental infection. In an other case, MENGELING *et al.* (1975) demonstrated masses of PPV-antigen in tissues of 6 mummified fetuses by means of immunofluorescent staining and, in addition, could isolate the virus in tissue culture. One normal appearing fetus had a HI-titer of 1:320. Since the gilt from which the fetuses were derived had no HI-antibody 67 days before farrowing but had developed a HI-titer of 1:1280 at the day of farrowing, infection with PPV during gestation was assumed. Finally, BACHMANN *et al.* (1975) reported on experimental *in utero* infection of pigs with PPV. Fetuses infected 35, 48, and 55 days of gestation died between 5 and 22 days after infection and appeared mummified. Virus was isolated from their organs and blood. Fetuses infected at 72, 94, and 105 days of gestation survived and developed high antibody titers *in utero*.

Attempts to characterize the etiologic agent of Aleutian disease of mink have now furnished strong evidence for this virus being a member of the *parvoviridae* (PORTER *et al.*, 1975). Virus particles adapted to growth in a feline kidney cell line were 24 nm in diameter and showed icosahedral symmetry. They proved resistant to the action of ether as well as to heating at 56° C for 30 minutes. In CsCl density gradients infective virions banded at a density of between 1.415 and 1.430 g/ml. Inhibition of viral replication in the presence of FUdR suggested the nucleic acid of the virus to be of DNA type. No antigenic relationship of Aleutian disease virus to 13 (!) other parvoviruses was detected.

References

1. ABINANTI, F. R., WARFIELD, M. S.: Recovery of a hemadsorbing virus (HADEN) from gastrointestinal tract of calves. Virology **14**, 288—289 (1961).
2. BABCOCK, V. I., SOUTHAM, C. M.: Stable cell line of rate nephroma in tissue culture. Proc. Soc. exp. Biol. (N.Y.) **124**, 217—219 (1967).
3. BACHMANN, P. A.: Vorkommen und Verbreitung von Picodna(parvo)-Virus beim Schwein. Zbl. Vet.-Med. **B16**, 341—345 (1969).
4. BACHMANN, P. A.: Parvoviren beim Schwein. Zbl. Vet.-Med. **B17**, 192—194(1970).
5. BACHMANN, P. A.: Properties of a bovine parvovirus. Zbl. Vet.-Med. **B18**, 80—85 (1971).
6. BAER, P. N., KILHAM, L.: Rat viruses and peridontal disease. I. The peridontium in mongoloid hamsters. Oral. Surg. **15**, 756—763 (1962).
7. BAER, P. N., KILHAM, L.: Rat viruses and peridontal disease. II. Onset and effect of age and time of inoculation. Oral. Surg. **15**, 1302—1311 (1962).
8. BAER, P. N., KILHAM, L.: Rat viruses and peridontal disease. III. The histopathology of early lesion in the first molar. Oral Surg. **17**, 116—124 (1964).
9. BAER, P. N., KILHAM, L.: Rat viruses and peridontal disease. IV. The aged hamster. Oral. Surg. **18**, 803—811 (1964).
10. BAER, P. N., KILHAM, L.: A comparison of the effects of four viruses on the peridontium of the Syrian hamster. Peridontol. **36**, 127—129 (1965).
11. BATES, R. C., STORZ, J.: Host cell range and growth characteristics of bovine parvovirus. Infect. Immun. **7**, 398—402 (1973).
12. BATES, R. C., STORZ, J., REED, D. E.: Isolation and characterization of bovine parvoviruses. J. infect. Dis. **126**, 531—536 (1972).
13. BENTINCK-SMITH, J.: Feline panleukopenia (feline infectious enteritis). A review of 574 cases. N. Amer. Vet. **30**, 379—384 (1949).
14. BERGS, V. V.: Leukemias induced in rats by mammary tumor extracts. J. nat. Cancer Inst. **38**, 481—490 (1967).
15. BERNHARD, W., KASTEN, F. H., CHANY, CH.: Etude cytochimique et ultrastructurale de cellules infectées par le virus K du rat et le virus H-1. C. R. Acad. Sci. (Paris) **257**, 1566—1569 (1963).
16. BERQUIST, K. R., MAYNARD, J. E., SHELLER, M., SCHABLE, C. A.: Comparative studies of hepatitis "candidate" agents and parvovirus in Detroit-6 cell cultures. J. infect. Dis. **126**, 203—205 (1972).
17. BINN, L. N., LAZAR, E. C., EDDY, G. A., KAJIMA, M.: Minute virus of canines. Bact. Proc. 68th Ann. Meeting Amer. Soc. Microbiol. **1967**, p. 161 (Abstract).
18. BINN, L. N., LAZAR, E. C., EDDY, G. A., KAJIMA, M.: Recovery and characterization of a minute virus of canines. Infect. Immun. **1**, 503—508 (1970).
19. BITTLE, J. L., EMERY, J. B., YORK, C. J., McMILLEN, J. K.: Comparative study of feline cytopathogenic viruses and feline panleukopenia virus. Amer. J. vet. Res. **22**, 374—378 (1961).
20. BOLIN, V. S.: The cultivation of panleukopenia virus in tissue culture. Virology **4**, 389—390 (1957).
21. BOUILLANT, A., HANSON, R. P.: Epizootiology of mink enteritis. III. Carrier state in mink. Canad. J. comp. Med. **29**, 183—189 (1965).
22. BRAILOVSKY, C.: Recherches sur le virus K du rat (Parvovirus Ratti). 1. Une méthode de titrage par plaques et son application a l'étude du cycle de multiplication du virus. Ann. Inst. Pasteur **110**, 49—59 (1966).
23. BRAILOVSKY, C., CHANY, C.: Un facteur produit par l'adénovirus 12 en culture cellulaire stimulant la multiplication du virus K du rat. C. R. Acad. Sci. (Paris) **260**, 2634—2637 (1965).
24. BREESE, S. S., JR., HOWATSON, A. F., CHANG, CH.: Isolation of virus-like particles associated with Kilham rat-virus infection of tissue cultures. Virology **24**, 598—603 (1964).
25. BURGER, D.: The relationship of mink virus enteritis to feline panleukopenia virus. Master Thesis, Washington State University, 1964.

26. BURGER, D., GORHAM, J. R., OTT, R. L.: Protection of cats against feline pan-
    leukopenia following mink enteritis virus vaccination. Small anim. Clin. **3**, 611
    (1963).
27. CARTWRIGHT, S. F., HUCK, R. A.: Viruses isolated in association with herd in-
    fertility, abortions, and still birth in pigs. Vet. Rec. **81**, 196—197 (1967).
28. CARTWRIGHT, S. F., LUCAS, M., HUCK, R. A.: A small hemagglutinating porcine
    DNA virus. I. Isolation and properties. J. comp. Path. **79**, 371—377 (1969).
29. CHANDRA, S., TOOLAN, H. W.: Electron microscopy of H-1 viruses. I. Morphology
    of the virus and a possible virus-host relationship. J. nat. Cancer Inst. **27**, 1405
    to 1449 (1961).
30. CHANY, C. H., BRAILOVSKY, C.: Les stimulons, facteurs antagonistes de l'inter-
    féron favorisant la multiplication intracellulaire des virus. C. R. Acad. Sci. (Paris)
    261, 4282—4285 (1965).
31. CHEONG, L., FOGH, J., BARCLAY, R. K.: Some properties of the H-1 virus and its
    nucleic acid. Fed. Proc. Abstracts **24**, 596 (1965).
32. CLARKE, D. H., CASALS, J.: Techniques for hemagglutination and hemagglutina-
    tion-inhibition with arthropod-borne viruses. Amer. J. trop. Med. Hyg. **7**, 561
    to 573 (1958).
33. COCHRAN, K. W., PAYNE, F. E.: Susceptibility of a strain of rat viruses to statolon
    and other virus inhibitors. Proc. Soc. exp. Biol. (N.Y.) **115**, 471—474 (1964).
34. COCUZZA, G., COSTARELLI, A.: Effect of coinfection with polyoma virus on multi-
    plication of picodnaviruses X-14 or H-1 in rat embryo cells. Boll. Ist. sieroter.
    milan. **48**, 301—304 (1969).
35. COCUZZA, G., MAIDA, A., NICOLETTI, G.: I Picodnavirus. Rassegna sintetica.
    Ann. Sclavo **9**, 367—380 (1967).
36. COCUZZA, G., RICCERI, G., DUSCIO, D., NICOLETTI, G.: L'attitiva timidina cinasica
    in cellule di embrione di ratto infettate con picodnavirus H-1 and X-14. Boll.
    Ist. sieroter. milan. **46**, 403—407 (1967).
37. COCUZZA, G., RUSSO, G.: Erythrocyte receptors in hemagglutination by picodna-
    viruses. Boll. Ist. sieroter. milan. **48**, 204—206 (1969).
38. COHEN, M. M., SHKLAR, G.: Deformities of the cranofacial and dental complex in
    the H-1 virus modified hamster. Oral. Surg. **17**, 533—541 (1964).
39. COLE, G. A., NATHANSON, N.: Immunofluorescent studies of the replication of rat
    virus (HER strain) in tissue culture. Acta virol. **13**, 515—520 (1969).
40. COLE, G. A., NATHANSON, N., RIVET, H.: Viral hemorrhagic encephalopathy of
    rats. II. Pathogenesis of central nervous system lesions. Amer. J. Epidem. **91**,
    339—350 (1970).
41. COLLMAN, R., STOLLER, A.: A survey of mongoloid births in Victoria, Australia
    1942—1957. Amer. J. publ. Hlth **52**, 813—829 (1962).
42. CRAWFORD, L. V.: A minute virus of mice. Virology **29**, 605—612 (1966).
43. CRAWFORD, L. V., FOLLET, E. A., BURDON, M. G., McGEOCH, D. J.: The DNA
    of a minute virus of mice. J. gen. Virol. **4**, 37—46 (1969).
44. CROGHAN, D. L., MATCHETT, A., KOSKI, T. A.: Isolation of porcine parvovirus
    from commercial trypsin. Appl. Microbiol. **26**, 431—433 (1973).
45. CROSS, S. S., PARKER, J. C.: Some antigenic relationships of the murine parvo-
    viruses: Minute virus of mice, rat, and H-1 virus. Proc. Soc. exp. Biol. (N.Y.)
    139, 105—108 (1972).
46. CSIZA, C. K., SCOTT, F. W., DE LAHUNTA, A., GILLESPIE, J. H.: Immune carrier
    state of feline panleukopenia virus-infected cats. Amer. J. vet. Res. **32**, 419—426
    (1971).
47. CSIZA, C. K., SCOTT, F. W., DE LAHUNTA, A., GILLESPIE, J. H.: Feline viruses.
    XIV. Transplacental infections in spontaneous panleukopenia of cats. Cornell
    Vet. **61**, 423—439 (1971).
48. DALLDORF, G.: Viruses and human cancer. Bull. N.Y. Acad. Med. **36**, 795—803
    (1960).
49. DALTON, A. J., KILHAM, L., ZEIGEL, R. F.: A comparison of polyoma "K", and
    Kilham rat viruses with the electron microscope. Virology **20**, 391—398 (1963).

50. DARBYSHIRE, J. H., ROBERTS, D. H.: Some respiratory virus and mycoplasma infections of animals. J. clin. Path., Suppl. 2, 61 (1968).
51. DAWE, C. J., KILHAM, L., MORGAN, W. D.: Intranuclear inclusions in tissue cultures infected with rat viruses. J. nat. Cancer Inst. 27, 221—235 (1961).
52. EL DADAH, A. N., NATHANSON, N., SMITH, K. O., MELBY, E. C.: Viral hemorrhagic encephalopathy of rats. Science 156, 392—394 (1964).
53. DEINHARDT, F., HOLMES, A. W., CAPPS, R. B., POPPER, H.: Studies on the transmission of human viral hepatitis to marmoset monkeys. I. Transmission of disease, serial passages and description of liver lesions. J. exp. Med. 125, 673—688 (1967).
54. DOBSON, P. R., HELLEINER, C. W.: A replicative form of the DNA of the minute virus of mice. Canad. J. Microbiol. 19, 35—41 (1973).
55. DUNNING, W. P., CURTIS, M. R.: A transplantable acute leukemia in an inbred line of rats. J. nat. Cancer Inst. 19, 845—852 (1957).
56. ENGLER, W. O., BAER, P. N., KILHAM, L.: Effects of rat virus on healing osseous wounds. Arch. Path. 82, 93—98 (1966).
57. FARELL, R. K., BURGER, D., HARTSOUGH, G. R., GORHAM, J. R.: Relationship of mink enteritis virus and feline panleukopenia virus: Rapid onset of mink virus enteritis virus protection after feline panleukopenia virus infection. Amer. J. vet. Res. 33, 2351—2352 (1972).
58. FEINSTONE, S. M., KAPIKIAN, A. Z., PURCELL, R. H.: Hepatitis A: Detection by immune electron microscopy of a virus-like antigen associated with acute illness. Nature (Lond.) 182, 1026—1028 (1973).
59. FEINSTONE, S. M., KAPIKIAN, A. Z., GERIN, J. L., PURCELL, R. H.: Buoyant density of the hepatitis A virus-like particles in cesium chloride. J. Virol. 13, 1412—1414 (1974).
60. FERM, V. H., KILHAM, L.: Rat virus (RV) infection in fetal and pregnant hamsters. Proc. Soc. exp. Biol. (N.Y.) 112, 623—626 (1963).
61. FERM, V. H., KILHAM, L.: Congenital anomalies induced in hamster embryos with H-1 virus. Science 148, 510—511 (1964).
62. FERM, V. H., KILHAM, L.: Skeletal studies of virus-induced dwarfism. Growth 29, 7—16 (1965).
63. FERM, V. H., KILHAM, L.: Histopathologic basis of the teratogenic effects of H-1 virus on hamster embryos. J. Embryol. exp. Morph. 13, 151—158 (1965).
64. FONG, C. K. Y., LEDINKO, N., TOOLAN, H. W.: Thymidine kinase activity and DNA synthesis in cells infected with the parvovirus H-1. Proc. Soc. exp. Biol. (N.Y.) 134, 1199—1202 (1970).
65. FONG, C. K. Y., TOOLAN, H. W., HOPKINS, M. S.: Effect of H-1 virus infection on RNA synthesis in NB cells. Proc. Soc. exp. Biol. (N.Y.) 135, 585—588 (1970).
66. FOWLER, E. H., ROHOVSKY, M. W.: Enzyme histochemistry of small intestine in germfree and specific pathogen-free cats inoculated with feline infectious enteritis (feline panleukopenia) virus. Amer. J. vet. Res. 31, 2055—2060 (1970).
67. FOWLER, E. A., ROHOVSKY, M. W.: Enzyme histochemistry of lymphoid tissues in germfree cats inoculated with feline infectious enteritis (feline panleukopenia) virus. Amer. J. vet. Res. 31, 2061—2069 (1970).
68. GALTON, M., KILHAM, L.: Chromosomes of "mongoloid" hamsters. Proc. Soc. exp. Biol. (N.Y.) 122, 18—22 (1966).
69. GAUTSCHI, M., SIEGL, G.: Structural proteins of parvovirus Lu III. Evidence for only two protein components within infectious virions. Arch. ges. Virusforsch. 43, 226—233 (1973).
70. GAUTSCHI, M., SIEGL, G., KRONAUER, G.: The multiplication of parvovirus Lu III in a synchronized culture system. IV. Association of viral structural polypeptides with the host cell chromatin. (In press, 1976.)
71. GAUTSCHI, M., SIEGL, G., TRACHSEL, H.: Erlaubt der Nachweis der Strukturproteine des Parvovirus Lu III in den Proteinfraktionen des Zellkerns Aussagen über die Vorgänge bei der Virusreifung? 5. Arbeitstag. Deutsche Ges. Hyg. Mikrobiologie Mainz, 1974. Abstr. in Zbl. Bakt. II. Abt. Ref. (1975).

72. GORHAM, J. R., HARTSOUGH, G. R.: Infectious enteritis of mink. J. Amer. vet. med. Ass. **126**, 467 (1955).
73. GORHAM, J. R., HARTSOUGH, G. R., BURGER, D., LUST, S., SATO, N.: The preliminary use of attenuated feline panleukopenia virus to protect cats against panleukopenia and mink against virus enteritis. Cornell Vet. **55**, 559—563 (1965).
74. GORHAM, J. R., HARTSOUGH, G. R., SATO, N., LUST, S.: Studies on cell culture-adapted feline panleukopenia virus—virus neutralization and antigenic extinction. Vet. Med. **61**, 35—40 (1966).
75. GREENE, E. L.: Ph. D. Thesis, Cornell University, Ithaca, N.Y., 1964.
76. GREENE, E. L.: Physical and chemical properties of H-1 virus. I. pH and heat stability of the hemagglutinating property. Proc. Soc. exp. Biol. (N.Y.) **118**, 973—975 (1975).
77. GREENE, E. L., KARASAKI, S.: Physical and chemical properties of H-1 virus. II. Partial purification. Proc. Soc. exp. Biol. (N.Y.) **119**, 918—922 (1965).
78. HALLAUER, C., KRONAUER, G.: Nachweis von Gelbfiebervirus-Hämagglutinin in menschlichen Explantaten. Arch. ges. Virusforsch. **10**, 267—287 (1960).
79. HALLAUER, C., KRONAUER, G.: Nachweis eines nicht identifizierten Hämagglutinins in menschlichen Tumorzellstämmen. Arch. ges. Virusforsch. **11**, 754 bis 756 (1962).
80. HALLAUER, C., KRONAUER, G.: Extraction of cell-associated virus without damage of the culture. Arch. ges. Virusforsch. **15**, 433—440 (1965).
81. HALLAUER, C., KRONAUER, G., SIEGL, G.: Parvoviruses as contaminants of permanent human cell lines. I. Virus isolations from 1960—1970. Arch. ges. Virusforsch. **35**, 80—90 (1971).
82. HALLAUER, C., SIEGL, G., KRONAUER, G.: Parvoviruses as contaminants of permanent human cell lines. III. The biologic properties of the isolated viruses. Arch. ges. Virusforsch. **38**, 366—382 (1972).
83. HAMMON, W. D., ENDERS, J. F.: A virus disease of cats, principally characterized by aleucocytosis, enteric lesions, and the presence of intranuclear inclusions bodies. J. exp. Med. **69**, 327—352 (1939).
84. HAMMON, W. D., ENDERS, J. F.: Further studies on the blood and the hemopoetic tissues in malignant panleukopenia of cats. J. exp. Med. **70**, 557—564 (1939).
85. HAMPTON, E. G.: Viral antigen in rat embryo in culture infected with H-1 virus isolated from transplantable human tumors. Cytochemical studies. Cancer Res. **24**, 1534—1543 (1964).
86. HAMPTON, E. G.: H-1 virus growth in synchronized rat embryo cells. Canad. J. Microbiol. **16**, 266—268 (1970).
87. HINDLE, E., FINDLAY, G. M.: Studies on feline distemper. J. comp. Path. **45**, 11 (1932).
88. HOGGAN, M. D.: Adenovirus-associated viruses. Progr. med. Virol. **12**, 211—239 (1970).
89. HOGGAN, M. D.: Small DNA viruses. In: Comparative Virology (MARAMOROSCH, K., KURSTAK, E., eds.). New York-London: Academic Press, 1971.
90. HORZINEK, M., UEBERSCHAER, S.: Charakterisierung eines Schweine-Adenovirus im Zusammenhang mit Untersuchungen über das Virus der europäischen Schweinepest. Arch. ges. Virusforsch. **18**, 406—421 (1966).
91. HORZINEK, M., MUSSGAY, M., MAESS, J., PETZOLDT, K.: Nachweis dreier Virusarten (Schweinepest-, Adeno-, Picodnavirus) in einem als cytopathogen bezeichneten Schweinepest-Virusstamm. Arch. ges. Virusforsch. **21**, 98—112 (1967).
92. HUYGELEN, C., PEETERMANS, J.: Isolation of a hemagglutinating picornavirus from primary swine kidney cell cultures. Arch. ges. Virusforsch. **20**, 260—262 (1967).
93. INABA, Y., KUROGI, H., TANAKA, Y., SATO, K., OMORI, T., ITO, Y.: A small hemagglutinating bovine DNA virus. I. Isolation and properties. Jap. J. vet. Sci. **33** (Suppl.), 188—189 (1971).
94. INABA, Y., KUROGI, H., TAKAHASHI, E., SATO, K., TANAKY, Y., GOTO, Y., OMORI, T., MATUMOTO, M.: Isolation and properties of bovine parvovirus type 1 from Japanese calves. Arch. ges. Virusforsch. **42**, 54—66 (1973).

95. INABA, Y., OMORI, T., KONO, M., ISHII, S., MATUMOTO, M.: A new serotype of bovine parvovirus. Jap. J. Microbiol. **17**, 85—86 (1973).

96. JAMISON, R. M., MAYOR, H. D.: Acridine orange staining of purified rat virus strain X-14. J. Bact. **90**, 1486—1488 (1965).

97. JOHNSON, R. H.: Isolation of a virus from a condition stimulating feline panleukopenia in a leopard. Vet. Rec. **76**, 1008—1012 (1964).

98. JOHNSON, R. H.: Feline panleukopenia. I. Identification of a virus associated with the syndrome. Res. Vet. Sci. **6**, 466—471 (1965).

99. JOHNSON, R. H.: Feline panleukopenia virus. II. Some features of the cytopathic effect in feline kidney monolayers. Res. Vet. Sci. **6**, 472—480 (1965).

100. JOHNSON, R. H.: Virus of feline panleukopenia. Nature (Lond.) **205**, 107 (1965).

101. JOHNSON, R. H.: Feline panleukopenia virus—*in vitro* comparison of strains with a mink enteritis virus. J. small Anim. Pract. **8**, 319—323 (1967).

102. JOHNSON, R. H.: Feline panleukopenia virus. IV. Methods for obtaining reproducible *in vitro* results. Res. Vet. Sci. **8**, 256—264 (1967).

103. JOHNSON, R. H.: A search for parvoviridae (Picodnaviridae). Vet. Rec. **84**, 19—20 (1969).

104. JOHNSON, R. H.: Feline panleukopenia. Vet. Rec. **84**, 338—340 (1969).

105. JOHNSON, R. H., COLLINGS, D. F.: Experimental infection of piglets and pregnant gilts with a parvovirus. Vet. Rec. **85**, 446—447 (1969).

106. JOHNSON, R. H., CRUICKSHANK, J. G.: Problems in classification of feline panleukopenia virus. Nature (Lond.) **212**, 622—623 (1966).

107. JOHNSON, R. H., MARGOLIS, G., KILHAM, L.: Identity of feline ataxia virus with feline panleukopenia virus. Nature (Lond.) **214**, 175—177 (1967).

108. JOHNSON, R. H., SIEGL, G., GAUTSCHI, M.: Characteristics of feline panleukopenia virus strains enabling definitive classification as parvoviruses. Arch. ges. Virusforsch. **46**, 315—324 (1974).

109. JOHNSON, F. B., HOGGAN, M. D.: Structural proteins of HADEN-virus. Virology **51**, 129—137 (1973).

110. JOHNSON, G. R., KOESTNER, A., ROHOVSKY, M. W.: Experimental feline infectious enteritis in the germfree cat. An electron microscopic study. Path. Vet. **4**, 275—288 (1967).

111. KAPIKIAN, A. Z., GERIN, J. L., WYATT, R. G., THORNHILL, T. S., CHANOCK, R. M.: Density in cesium chloride of the 27 nm "8FIIa" particle associated with acute infectious nonbacterial gastroenteritis: Determination by ultracentrifugation and immune electron microscopy. Proc. Soc. exp. Biol. (N.Y.) **142**, 874—877 (1973).

112. KAPIKIAN, A. Z., WYATT, R. G., DOBIN, R., THORNHILL, T. S., KALICA, A. R., CHANOCK, R. M.: Visualization by immune electron microscopy of a 27 nm particle associated with acute infectious nonbacterial gastroenteritis. J. Virol. **10**, 1075—1081 (1972).

113. KARASAKI, S.: Size and ultrastructure of the H-viruses as determined with the use of specific antibodies. J. Ultrastruct. Res. **16**, 109—122 (1966).

114. KARASAKI, S., TOOLAN, H. W., USATEGUI-GOMEZ, M.: A human placental fluid inhibitor to hemagglutination by H-1 and HB viruses. II. Electron microscope studies. Proc. Soc. exp. Biol. (N.Y.) **120**, 391—394 (1965).

115. KIKUTH, W., GOENNERT, R., SCHWEIKERT, M.: Infektiöse Aleukozytose der Katzen. Zbl. Bakt. I. Abt. Orig. **146**, 1—17 (1940).

116. KILHAM, L.: Rat virus (RV) infections in the hamster. Proc. Soc. exp. Biol. (N.Y.) **106**, 825—829 (1961).

117. KILHAM, L.: Mongolism associated with rat virus (RV) infection in hamsters. Virology **13**, 141—143 (1961).

118. KILHAM, L.: Viruses of laboratory and wild rats. Nat. Cancer Inst. Monogr. No. **20**, 117—135 (1966).

119. KILHAM, L., FERM, V. H.: Rat virus (RV) infection in pregnant, fetal, and newborn rats. Proc. Soc. exp. Biol. (N.Y.) **117**, 874—879 (1964).

120. KILHAM, L., MOLONEY, V. B.: Association of rat virus and Moloney leukemia virus in tissues of inoculated rats. J. nat. Cancer Inst. **32**, 523—531 (1964).

121. KILHAM, L., MARGOLIS, G.: Cerebellar ataxia in hamsters inoculated with rat virus. Science **143**, 1047—1048 (1964).
122. KILHAM, L., MARGOLIS, G.: Cerebellar disease in cats induced by inoculation of rat virus. Science **148**, 244—245 (1965).
123. KILHAM, L., MARGOLIS, G.: Viral etiology of spontaneous ataxia of cats. Amer. J. Path. **48**, 991—1011 (1966).
124. KILHAM, L., MARGOLIS, G.: Spontaneous hepatitis and cerebellar hypoplasia in suckling rats due to congenital infection with rat virus. Amer. J. Path. **49**, 457 to 475 (1966).
125. KILHAM, L., MARGOLIS, G.: Transplacental infection of rats and hamsters induced by oral and parenteral inoculations of H-1 and rat viruses (RV). Teratology **2**, 111—123 (1969).
126. KILHAM, L., MARGOLIS, G.: Pathogenicity of a minute virus of mice (MVM) for rats, mice, and hamsters. Proc. Soc. exp. Biol. (N.Y.) **133**, 1447—1452 (1970).
127. KILHAM, L., MARGOLIS, G.: Fetal infections of hamsters, rats, and mice induced with the minute virus of mice (MVM). Teratology **4**, 43—61 (1971).
128. KILHAM, L., MARGOLIS, G., COLBY, E. D.: Congenital infections of cats and ferrets by feline panleukopenia viruses manifested by cerebellar hypoplasia. Lab. Invest. **17**, 465—480 (1967).
129. KILHAM, L., MARGOLIS, G., COLBY, E. D.: Enhanced proliferation of H-1 virus in livers of rats infected with *Cysticercus fasciolaris*. J. infect. Dis. **121**, 648—652 (1970).
130. KILHAM, L., MARGOLIS, G., COLBY, E. D.: Cerebellar ataxia and its congenital transmission in cats by feline panleukopenia virus. J. Amer. med. Ass. **158**, 888 to 901 (1971).
131. KILHAM, L., OLIVIER, L. J.: A latent virus of rats isolated in tissue culture. Virology **7**, 428—437 (1959).
132. KIM, Y. B., BRADLEY, S. G., WARSON, D. W.: Development of immunoglobulins in germfree and conventional colostrum-deprived piglets. Fed. Proc. **23**, 346 (1964).
133. KING, D. A., CROGHAN, D. L.: Immunofluorescence of feline panleukopenia virus in cell culture: Determination of immunological status of felines by serum neutralization. Canad. J. comp. Med. **29**, 85—89 (1965).
134. KLEINSCHMIDT, A., ZAHN, R. K.: Über Deoxyribonukleinsäure-Molekeln in Protein-Mischfilmen. Z. Naturforsch. **14 b**, 770 (1959).
135. KNOX, B.: Virus enteritis of mink in Denmark. N. vet. Med. **12**, 145—169 (1960).
136. KONGSVIK, J. R., GIERTHY, J. F., RHODE, S. L.: Replication process of the parvovirus H-1. IV. H-1 specific proteins synthesized in synchronized human NB kidney cells. J. Virol. **14**, 1600—1603 (1974).
137. KONGSVIK, J. R., SINGER, I. I., TOOLAN, H. W.: Studies on the red cell and antibody reactive sites of the parvovirus H-1: Effect of fixatives. Proc. Soc. exp. Biol. (N.Y.) **145**, 763—770 (1974).
138. KONGSVIK, J. R., TOOLAN, H. W.: Capsid components of the parvovirus H-1. Proc. Soc. exp. Biol. (N.Y.) **139**, 1202—1205 (1972).
139. KONGSVIK, J. R., TOOLAN, H. W.: Effect of proteolytic enzymes on the hemagglutinating property of the parvoviruses H-1, H-3, and RV. Proc. Soc. exp. Biol. (N.Y.) **140**, 140—144 (1972).
140. KURSTAK, E.: Small DNA densonucleosis virus (DNC). Advanc. Virus Res. **17**, 207—241 (1972).
141. AL-LAMI, F., LEDINKO, N., TOOLAN, H. W.: Electron microscope study of human NB and SMH cells infected with the parvovirus H-1. Involvement of the nucleolus. J. gen. Virol. **5**, 485—492 (1969).
142. LAWRENCE, J. S., SYVERTON, J. T.: Spontaneous agranulocytosis in the cat. Proc. Soc. exp. Biol. (N.Y.) **38**, 914—918 (1938).
143. LAWRENCE, J. S., SYVERTON, J. T., SHAW, J. S., JR., SMITH, F. P.: Infectious feline agranulocytosis. Amer. J. Path. **16**, 333—354 (1940).

144. LAWRENCE, J. S., SYVERTON, J. T., ACKART, R. J., ADAMS, W. S., ERVIN, D. M., HASKINS, A. L., JR., SOUNDERS, R. H., JR., STRINGFELLOW, M. B., WETRICK, R. M.: The viruses of infectious feline agranulocytosis. II. Immunological relation to other viruses. J. exp. Med. **77**, 57—64 (1943).

145. LEASURE, E. E., LIENHARDT, H. F., TABERNER, F. R.: Feline infectious enteritis. N. Amer. Vet. **15**, 30—44 (1934).

146. LEDINKO, N.: Plaque assay of the effects of cytosine arabinoside and 5-iodo-deoxyuridine on the synthesis of H-1 virus particles. Nature (Lond.) **214**, 1346 to 1347 (1967).

147. LEDINKO, N., HOPKINS, S., TOOLAN, H. W.: Relationship between potentiation of H-1 growth by human adenovirus 12 and inhibition of the "helper" adenovirus by H-1. J. gen. Virol. **5**, 19—31 (1969).

148. LEDINKO, N., TOOLAN, H. W.: Human adenovirus type 12 as a "helper" for growth of H-1 virus. J. Virol. **2**, 155—156 (1968).

149. LEDINKO, N., TOOLAN, H. W.: Relationship between induction of thymidine kinase and potentiation or growth of H-1 virus by human adenovirus 12. J. gen. Virol. **7**, 263—266 (1970).

150. LUCAS, A. M., RISER, W. H.: Intranuclear inclusions in panleukopenia of cats. A correlation with the pathogenesis of the disease and comparison with inclusions of herpes, B-virus, yellow fever, and burns. Amer. J. Path. **21**, 435 (1945).

151. LUM, G. S.: Serological studies of rat viruses in relation to tumors. Oncology **24**, 335—343 (1970).

152. LUM, G. S.: In vitro studies of rat viruses. I. Effects of long-term culture. Oncology **24**, 401—415 (1970).

153. LUM, G. S.: In vitro studies of rat viruses. Effects of heat, X-irradiation, and carcinogenic drugs. Oncology **24**, 416—430 (1970).

154. LUM, G. S., SCHREINER, A. W.: Study of a virus isolated from a chloroleukemic Wistar rat. Cancer Res. **23**, 1742—1747 (1963).

155. LUST, S. J., GORHAM, J. R., SATO, N.: The occurrence of intranuclear inclusions in cell cultures infected with infectious feline panleukopenia virus. Amer. J. vet. Res. **26**, 1163—1166 (1965).

156. MACCHIAVELLO, A., BEZERRA CONTINHO, A.: Epizootias felinas do nordeste do Brasil. Adeno-myelo-enterose especifica por virus fultravel. Brasil-méd. **54**, 113 to 118 (1940).

157. MAHNEL, H.: Virus-like particles from hog cholera infected tissue cultures and demonstrated in the electron microscope. "FAO/OIE Meeting on hog cholera and African swine fever", Rome, Italy, June 1965.

158. MAHNEL, H., BIBRACK, B.: Isolierung von Adenoviren aus Zellkulturen von Nieren normaler Schlachtschweine. Zbl. Bakt. I. Abt. Orig. **199**, 329—338 (1966).

159. MARGOLIS, G., KILHAM, L.: Rat virus, an agent with an affinity for the dividing cell. In: Slow, Latent, and Temperate Virus Infections. NINDB Monograph **2**, 361—367 (1965).

160. MARGOLIS, G., KILHAM, L., RUFFALO, P. R.: Rat disease, and an experimental model of neonatal hepatitis. Exp. molec. Path. **8**, 1—20 (1968).

161. MATSUO, Y., SPENCER, H. J.: Studies on the infectivity of rat virus (RV) in BALB/c mice. Proc. Soc. exp. Biol. (N.Y.) **130**, 294—299 (1969).

162. MAY, P., NIVELEAU, A., BERGER, G., BRAILOVSKY, C.: Recherches' sur le DNA du virus K du rat (Parvovirus Ratti). J. molec. Biol. **27**, 603—614 (1967).

163. MAY, P., MAY, E.: The DNA of Kilham rat virus. J. gen. Virol. **6**, 437—439 (1970).

164. MAYNARD, J. E., BRADLEY, D. W., GRAVELLE, C. R., HORNBECK, C. L., COOK, E. H.: Virus-like particles in hepatitis A. Lancet **7890**, 1207 (1974).

165. MAYOR, H. D., DIWAN, A. R.: Studies on acridine orange staining of two purified RNA viruses: Poliovirus and tobacco mosaic virus. Virology **14**, 74—82 (1961).

166. MAYOR, H. D., HILL, N. O.: Acridine orange staining of a single-stranded DNA-bacteriophage. Virology **14**, 264—266 (1961).

167. MAYOR, H. D., ITO, M.: The early detection of picodnavirus X-14 by immuno-fluorescence. Proc. Soc. exp. Biol. (N.Y.) **129**, 684—686 (1968).

168. MAYOR, H. D., JORDAN, E. L.: Electron microscopic study of the rodent "Picodna-virus" X-14. Exp. molec. Path. **5**, 580—589 (1966).
169. MAYOR, H. D., MELNICK, J. C.: Small deoxyribonucleic acid containing viruses (picodnavirus group). Nature (Lond.) **210**, 331—332 (1966).
170. MAYR, A., BACHMANN, P. A., SHEFFY, B. E., SIEGL, G.: Electron optical and buoyant density studies of hog cholera virus. Arch. ges. Virusforsch. **21**, 113—119 (1967).
171. MAYR, A., BACHMANN, P. A., SIEGL, G., SHEFFY, B. E.: Characterization of a small porcine DNA virus. Arch. ges. Virusforsch. **25**, 38—51 (1968).
172. MAYR, A., MAHNEL, H.: Züchtung von Schweinepestvirus in Schweinenieren-Kulturen mit cytopathogenem Effekt. Zbl. Bakt. I. Abt. Orig. **195**, 157—166 (1964).
173. MAYR, A., MAHNEL, H.: Weitere Untersuchungen über die Züchtung von Schweine-pestvirus in Zellkulturen mit cytopathogenem Effekt. Zbl. Bakt. I. Abt. Orig. **199**, 399—407 (1966).
174. McGEOCH, D. J., CRAWFORD, L. V., FOLLETT, E. A. C.: The DNA's of three parvoviruses. J. gen. Virol. **6**, 33—40 (1970).
175. McPHERSON, J. W.: Feline enteritis virus: Its transmission to mink under natural and experimental conditions. Canad. comp. Med. **20**, 197—202 (1956).
176. MELNICK, J. L., BOUCHER, D. W., CRASKE, J., BOGGS, J.: Properties of a virus isolated from patients with MS-1 infectious hepatitis. J. infect. Dis. **124**, 76—85 (1971).
177. MENGELING, W. L.: Porcine parvovirus: Properties and prevalence of a strain isolated in the United States. Amer. J. vet. Res. **33**, 2239—2248 (1972).
178. MOHANTY, S. B., BACHMANN, P. A.: Susceptibility of fertilized mouse eggs to minute virus of mice. Infect. Immun. **9**, 762—763 (1974).
179. MOORE, A. E.: Relationship between H-1, H-3, and RV viruses. Proc. Amer. Ass. Cancer Res. **3**, 345 (1962).
180. MOORE, A. E.: Characteristics of certain viruses isolated from transplantable tumors. Virology **18**, 182—191 (1962).
181. MOORE, A. E.: Fetal infection of A×C rats with H-viruses. Proc. Amer. Ass. Cancer Res. **4**, 45 (1963).
182. MOORE, A. E., NICASTRI, A. D.: Lethal infection and pathological findings in A×C rats inoculated with H-virus and RV. J. nat. Cancer Inst. **35**, 937—947 (1965).
183. MONIF, G. R., SEVER, J. L., COCHRAN, W. D.: The H-1 and RV-viruses and preg-nancy: Serological studies of certain groups of pregnant women. J. Pediat. **67**, 253—256 (1965).
184. MYERS, W. L., ALBERTS, J. C., BRANDLY, C. A.: Certain characteristics of the virus of infectious enteritis of mink and observations on pathogenesis of the disease. Canad. J. comp. Med. **23**, 283 (1959).
185. MYERS, W. L., FRITZ, T. E.: Histopathologic changes in virus enteritis of mink. Canad. J. comp. Med. **23**, 246 (1959).
186. NATHANSON, N., COLE, G. A., SANTOS, G. W., SQUIRE, R. A., SMITH, K. O.: Viral hemorrhagic encephalopathy of rats. I. Isolation, identification, and properties of the HER strain of rat virus. Amer. J. Epidem. **91**, 328—338 (1970).
187. NEWBORNE, J. W., JOHNSTON, R. V., ROBINSON, V. B.: Studies on clinical and histopathological aspects of feline panleukopenia (Infectious Enteritis). South-West Vet. **10**, 111—118 (1957).
188. NEWMAN, S. J., McCALLIN, P. F., SEVER, J. L.: Attempts to isolate H-1 virus from spontaneous human abortions: A negative report. Teratology **3**, 279—281 (1970).
189. NICHOLSON, B., HETTRICK, F. M.: Host influence on the antigenic composition of the Kilham rat virus. J. Virol. **4**, 619—625 (1969).
190. NICOLETTI, G., CASTRO, A., RUSSO, G., COCUZZA, G.: Citopatologia da picodna-virus (RV, H-1, X-14) in cellule di embrione di ratto. Ann. Sclavo **11**, 188—201 (1969).

191. Novotny, J. F., Hetrick, F. M.: Pathogenesis and transmission of Kilham rat virus infection in rats. Infect. Immun. **2**, 298—303 (1970).
192. O'Reilly, K. J.: Determination of an optimal dilution of virulent feline infectious enteritis (panleukopenia) virus for challenge purposes. J. Hyg. (Lond.) **68**, 549 to 556 (1970).
193. O'Reilly, K. J., Peterson, J. S., Harriss, S. T.: The persistence in kittens of maternal antibody to feline infectious enteritis (panleukopenia). Vet. Rec. **84**, 376—378 (1969).
194. O'Reilly, K. J., Whitaker, A. M.: The development of feline cell lines for the growth of feline infectious enteritis (panleukopenia) virus. J. Hyg. (Lond.) **67**, 115—124 (1969).
195. Parker, J. C., Collins, M. J., Cross, S. S., Rowe, W. P.: Minute virus of mice: Prevalence, epidemiology, and occurrence as a contaminant of transplanted tumors. J. nat. Cancer Inst. **45**, 305—310 (1970).
196. Parker, J. C., Cross, S. S., Collins, M. C., Rowe, W. P.: Minute virus of mice: Procedures for quantitation and detection. J. nat. Cancer Inst. **45**, 297—303 (1970).
197. Payne, F. E., Beals, T. F., Preston, R. E.: Morphology of a small DNA-virus. Virology **23**, 109—113 (1964).
198. Payne, F. E., Shellaberger, C. J., Schmidt, R. W.: A virus from mammary tissue of rats treated with X-rays or methylcholanthrene. Proc. Amer. Ass. Cancer Res. **4**, 51 (1963).
199. Poole, G. M.: Stability of a modified, live panleukopenia virus stored in liquid phase. Appl. Microbiol. **24**, 663—664 (1972).
200. Portella, O. B.: Hemadsorption and related studies on the hamster-osteolytic viruses. Arch. ges. Virusforsch. **14**, 277—305 (1964).
201. Polson, A., van Regenmortel, M. H. V.: A new method for determination of sedimentation constants of viruses. Virology **15**, 397—403 (1961).
202. Provost, P. J., Ittensohn, O. L., Villarejos, V. R., Arguedas, G., Hilleman, M. R.: Etiologic relationship of marmoset-propagated CR 326 hepatitis A virus to hepatitis in man. Proc. Soc. exp. Biol. (N.Y.) **142**, 1257—1267 (1973).
203. Rabson, A. S., Kilham, L., Kirschstein, R. L.: Intranuclear inclusions in *rattus* (Mastomys) *natalensis* infected with rat virus. J. nat. Cancer Inst. **27**, 1217 to 1223 (1961).
204. Reynolds, H. A.: Some clinical and hematological features of virus enteritis of mink. Canad. J. comp. Med. **33**, 155—159 (1969).
205. Rhode, S. L.: Replication process of parvovirus H-1: I. Kinetics in a parasynchronous cell system. J. Virol. **11**, 856—861 (1973).
206. Rhode, S. L.: Replication process of parvovirus H-1: II. Isolation and characterization of H-1 replicative form DNA. J. Virol. **13**, 400—410 (1974a).
207. Rhode, S. L.: Replication process of parvovirus H-1: III. Factors affecting RF DNA synthesis. J. Virol. **14**, 791—801 (1974b).
208. Riser, W. H.: Infectious panleukopenia of cats. N. Amer. Vet. **24**, 293—299 (1943).
209. Robey, R. E., Woodman, D. R., Hetrick, F. M.: Studies on the natural infection of rats with the Kilham rat virus. Amer. J. Epidem. **88**, 139—143 (1968).
210. Robinson, D. M., Hetrick, F. M.: Single-stranded DNA from the Kilham rat virus. J. gen. Virol. **4**, 269—281 (1969).
211. Rohovsky, M. W., Griesemer, R. A.: Experimental feline infectious enteritis in the cat. Path. Vet. **4**, 391—410 (1967).
212. Rose, J. A.: Parvovirus reproduction. In: Comprehensive Virology (Fraenkel-Conrat, H., Wagner, R., eds.). New York: Plenum Publishing Corp., 1975.
213. Ruffalo, P. R., Margolis, G., Kilham, L.: The induction of hepatitis by prior partial hepatectomy in resistant adult rats injected with H-1 virus. Amer. J. Path. **49**, 795—824 (1966).
214. Salzman, L. A.: DNA polymerase activity associated with purified Kilham rat virus. Nature (Lond.) **231**, 174—176 (1971).
215. Salzman, L. A., Jori, L. A.: Characterization of the Kilham rat virus. J. Virol. **5**, 114—122 (1970).

216. SALZMAN, L. A., WHITE, W. L.: Structural proteins of Kilham rat virus. Biochem. biophys. Res. Commun. **41**, 1551—1556 (1970).

217. SALZMAN, L. A., WHITE, W.: *In vivo* conversion of the single-stranded DNA of the Kilham rat virus to a double-stranded form. J. Virol. **11**, 299—305 (1973).

218. SALZMAN, L. A., WHITE, W. L., KAKEFUDA, T.: Linear, single-stranded DNA isolated from Kilham rat virus. J. Virol. **7**, 830—835 (1971).

219. SALZMAN, L. A., WHITE, W. L., McKERLIE, L.: Growth characteristics of Kilham rat virus and its effect on cellular macromolecular synthesis. J. Virol. **10**, 573 to 577 (1972).

220. SCHAFFER, F. L., SCHWERDT, C. E.: Purification and properties of poliovirus. Advanc. Virus Res. **6**, 159—204 (1959).

221. SCHILDKRAUT, C. L., MARMUR, J., DOTY, P.: Determination of base composition of deoxyribonucleic acid from its buoyant density in CsCl. J. molec. Biol. **4**, 430 to 443 (1962).

222. SCHOFIELD, F. W.: Virus enteritis in mink. N. Amer. Vet. **30**, 651 (1949).

223. SCOTT, F. W., CSIZA, C. K., GILLESPIE, J. H.: Feline viruses. IV. Isolation and characterization of feline panleukopenia virus in tissue culture and comparison of cytopathogenicity with feline picornavirus, herpesvirus, and reovirus. Cornell Vet. **60**, 165—183 (1970a).

224. SCOTT, F. W., CSIZA, C. K., GILLESPIE, J. H.: Feline viruses. V. Serum-neutralization test for feline panleukopenia. Cornell Vet. **60**, 183 (1970b).

225. SCOTT, F. W., CSIZA, C. K., GILLESPIE, J. H.: Maternally derived immunity to feline panleukopenia. J. Amer. vet. med. Ass. **156**, 439—453 (1970c).

226. SIEGL, G.: Parvoviruses as contaminants of permanent human cell lines. V. The nucleic acid of KBSH-virus. Arch. ges. Virusforsch. **37**, 267—274 (1972).

227. SIEGL, G.: Physicochemical characteristics of the DNA of parvovirus LuIII. Arch. ges. Virusforsch. **43**, 334—344 (1973).

228. SIEGL, G.: Lineare Doppelstränge und verzweigte Moleküle als Zwischenformen in der Synthese der einsträngigen, linearen DNS eines Parvovirus. 32. Jahresvers. Schweizer. Mikrobiol. Ges., Nyon 1973. Abstr. in Path. et Microbiol. (Basel) **40**, 202—203 (1974).

229. SIEGL, G., GAUTSCHI, M.: The multiplication of parvovirus LuIII in a synchronized culture system. I. Optimum conditions for virus replication. Arch. ges. Virusforsch. **40**, 105—118 (1973).

230. SIEGL, G., GAUTSCHI, M.: The multiplication of parvovirus LuIII in a synchronized culture system. II. Biochemical characteristics of virus replication. Arch. ges. Virusforsch. **40**, 119—127 (1973).

231. SIEGL, G., GAUTSCHI, M.: The multiplication of parvovirus LuIII in a synchronized culture system. III. Replication of viral DNA. J. Virol. (1976).

232. SIEGL, G., HALLAUER, C., NOVAK, A., KRONAUER, G.: Parvoviruses as contaminants of permanent human cell lines. II. Physicochemical properties of the isolated viruses. Arch. ges. Virusforsch. **35**, 91—103 (1971).

233. SIEGL, G., HALLAUER, C., NOVAK, A.: Parvoviruses as contaminants of permanent human cell lines. IV. Multiplication of KBSH-virus in KB cells. Arch. ges. Virusforsch. **36**, 351—362 (1972).

234. SINSHEIMER, R. L., A single-stranded deoxyribonucleic acid from bacteriophage ΦX 174. J. molec. Biol. **1**, 43—53 (1959).

235. SOIKE, K. F., IATROPOULIS, M., SIEGL, G.: Infection of newborn and fetal hamsters induced by inoculation of LuIII parvovirus. Arch. Virol. (1976) in press.

236. SPAHN, G. J., MOHANTY, S. B., HETRICK, F. M.: Characteristics of hemadsorbing enteric (HADEN) virus. Canad. J. Microbiol. **12**, 653—661 (1966).

237. SPAHN, G. J., MOHANTY, S. B., HETRICK, F. M.: Experimental infection of calves with hemadsorbing enteric (HADEN) virus. Cornell Vet. **56**, 377—386 (1966).

238. SPENCER, H. J.: Recovery of rat virus from a series of chemically induced rat leukemia. Proc. Amer. Ass. Cancer Res. **8**, 62 (1967).

239. STORZ, J., BATES, R. C.: Parvovirus infections in calves. J. Amer. vet. med. Ass. **163**, 884—886 (1973).

240. Storz, J., Bates, R. C., Warren, G. S., Howard, T. H.: Distribution of antibodies against bovine parvovirus 1 in cattle and other animal species. Amer. J. vet. Res. **33**, 269—272 (1972).

241. Storz, J., Warren, G. S.: Effect of antimetabolites and actinomycin D on the replication of HADEN, a bovine parvovirus. Arch. ges. Virusforsch. **30**, 271—274 (1970).

242. Studdert, M. J., Peterson, J. E.: Some properties of feline panleukopenia virus. Arch. ges. Virusforsch. **42**, 346—354 (1973).

243. Syverton, J. T., Lawrence, J. S., Ackert, R. J., Adams, W. S., Ervin, D. M., Maskins, A. L., Saunders, R. H., Stringfellow, M. B., Wetrick, R. M.: The virus of infectious feline agranulocytosis. I. Characters of the virus: Pathogenicity. J. exp. Med. **77**, 41—56 (1943).

244. Tattersall, P.: Replication of parvovirus MVM. I. Dependence of virus-multiplication and plaque formation on cell growth. J. Virol. **10**, 586—590 (1972).

245. Tattersall, P., Crawford, L. V., Shatkin, A. J.: Replication of the parvovirus MVM. II. Isolation and characterization of intermediates in the replication of the viral deoxyribonucleic acid. J. Virol. **12**, 1446—1456 (1973).

246. Tennant, R. W., Hand, R. E.: Requirement of cellular synthesis for Kilham rat virus. Virology **42**, 1054—1063 (1970).

247. Tennant, R. W., Layman, K. R., Hand, R. E.: Effect of cell physiological state on infection by rat virus. J. Virol. **4**, 872—878 (1969).

248. Toolan, H. W.: Production of a "mongolian-idiot" like abnormality in hamsters. Fed. Proc. **19**, 208 (1960).

249. Toolan, H. W.: Experimental production of mongoloid hamsters. Science **131**, 1446—1448 (1960).

250. Toolan, H. W.: A virus associated with transplantable human tumors. Bull. N.Y. Acad. Med. **37**, 305—310 (1961).

251. Toolan, H. W.: Studies on a viral agent associated with human tissues. Proc. Amer. Ass. Cancer Res. **3**, 273—274 (1961).

252. Toolan, H. W.: Studies on H-viruses. Proc. Amer. Ass. Cancer Res. **5**, 64 (1964).

253. Toolan, H. W.: H-1 virus in the adult hamster. Proc. Soc. exp. Biol. (N.Y.) **119**, 715—717 (1965).

254. Toolan, H. W.: Susceptibility of the rhesus monkey (Macaca mulatta) to H-1 virus. Nature (Lond.) **209**, 833—834 (1966).

255. Toolan, H. W.: Lack of oncogenic effect of the H-viruses for hamsters. Nature (Lond.) **214**, 1036 (1967).

256. Toolan, H. W.: Agglutination of the H-viruses with various types of red blood cells. Proc. Soc. exp. Biol. (N.Y.) **124**, 144—146 (1967).

257. Toolan, H. W.: The picodnaviruses: H, RV, and AAV. Int. Rev. exp. Path. **6**, 135—180 (1968).

258. Toolan, H. W., Buttle, G. A. H., Kay, H. E. M.: Isolation of the H-1 and H-3 viruses directly from human embryos. Proc. Amer. Ass. Cancer Res. **5**, 64 (1964).

259. Toolan, H. W., Dalldorf, G., Barclay, M., Chandra, S., Moore, A. E.: An unidentified filtrable agent isolated from transplanted human tumors. Proc. nat. Acad. Sci. (Wash.) **46**, 1256 (1960).

260. Toolan, H. W., Ledinko, N.: Growth and cytopathogenicity of H-viruses in human and simian cell cultures. Nature (Lond.) **208**, 812—813 (1965).

261. Toolan, H. W., Sounders, E. L., Greene, E. L., Fabricio, D. P. A.: Further studies on the electron microscopy of the H-1 virus. Virology **22**, 286—288 (1964).

262. Toolan, H. W., Sounders, E. L., Southam, C. M., Moore, A. E., Levin, A. G.: H-1 virus viremia in the human. Proc. Soc. exp. Biol. (N.Y.) **119**, 711—715 (1965).

263. Tromans, W. J., Horns, R. W.: The structure of bacteriophage ΦX 174. Virology **15**, 1—7 (1961).

264. Urbain, A.: Contribution à l'étude de la gastro-entérite infectieuse des chats. Ann. Inst. Pasteur **51**, 202—214 (1933).

265. Urbano, P.: Isolamento di un virus polio tipo 2 da un lotto di tripsina commerciale. Boll. Ist. sieroter. milan. **48**, 443—448 (1969).

266. USATEGUI-GOMEZ, M.: A human placental fluid inhibitor to hemagglutination by H-1 and HB viruses. Proc. Soc. exp. Biol. (N.Y.) **120**, 385—390 (1965).
267. USATEGUI-GOMEZ, M., MORGAN, D. F.: Further purification of a human placental inhibitor to hemagglutination by H-1 virus. Proc. Soc. exp. Biol. (N.Y.) **127**, 244 to 251 (1968).
268. USATEGUI-GOMEZ, M., TOOLAN, H. W., LEDINKO, N., AL-LAMI, F., HOPKINS, M. S.: Single-stranded DNA from the parvovirus H-1. Virology **39**, 617—621 (1969).
269. VASQUEZ, C., BRAILOVSKY, C.: Purification and fine structure of Kilham's rat virus. Exp. molec. Path. **4**, 130—140 (1965).
270. VERGE, J., CHRISTOFERONI, N.: La gastro-entérite infectieuse des chats est-elle due à un virus filtrable? C. R. Soc. Biol. (Paris) **99**, 312—314 (1928).
271. VINCENT, J.: Isolement en Algérie de quatre souches de parvovirus bovis. Ann. Inst. Pasteur **121**, 811—814 (1971).
272. WHELLY, J. M.: Rat virus nucleic acid. Biochem. J. **94**, 10 (1965).
273. WHITMAN, J. E., HETRICK, F. M.: Purification of the Kilham rat virus. Appl. Microbiol. **15**, 62—66 (1967).
274. WILLS, C. G.: Notes on infectious enteritis of mink and its relationship to feline enteritis. Canad. J. comp. Med. **16**, 419—420 (1952).
275. WILLS, C. G.: Infectious enteritis of mink. Fur Trade J. Canada **30**, 10—29 (1953).
276. WILLS, C. G., BELCHER, J.: The prevention of virus enteritis of mink with commercial feline panleukopenia vaccine. J. Amer. vet. med. Ass. **128**, 559—563 (1956).
277. WOZNIAK, J., HETRICK, F.: Persistent infection of a rat nephrome cell line with Kilham rat virus. J. Virol. **4**, 313—314 (1969).
278. ZHDANOV, V. M., MEREKALOVA, Z. I.: Isolation of a virus from connective tissue of carcinogen-treated rats. Vop. Virus. **7**, 339—342 (1962).
279. ZSCHOKKE, E.: Über coli-bacilläre Infektionen. Schweiz. Arch. Tierheilk. **42**, 20—30 (1900).
280. ZWILLENBERG, L. O., HALLAUER, C.: An unidentified hemagglutinin from human tumor tissue cultures. Arch. ges. Virusforsch. **12**, 393—403 (1962).

References to Addendum

1 A. BACHMANN, P. A., SHEFFY, B. E., VAUGHAN, J. T.: Experimental *in utero* infection of fetal pigs with porcine parvovirus. Infect. Immun. **12**, 455—460 (1975).
2 A. BACHMANN, P. A., HOGGAN, M. D., MELNICK, J. L., PEREIRA, H. G., VAGO, C.: *Parvoviridae.* Intervirology **5**, 83—92 (1975).
3 A. BATES, R. C., STORZ, J., DOUGHRI, A. M.: Morphogenesis of bovine parvovirus and associated cellular changes. Exp. molec. Path. **20**, 208—215 (1974).
4 A. BOURGIGNON, G. J., TATTERSALL, P. J., WARD, D. C.: The DNA of Minute Virus of Mice: A single-stranded genome with a 5'-terminal hairpin duplex. Abstr. Third Int. Congr. Virology, Madrid, p. 181 (1975).
5 A. CLINTON, G. M., HAYASHI, M.: The parvovirus MVM: Particles with altered structural proteins. Virology **66**, 261—267 (1975).
6 A. HENRY, C. J., DIARIO, A. F.: Induction of hepatitis in adult Syrian hamsters by H-1 virus. Proc. Soc. exp. Biol. (N.Y.) **149**, 23—28 (1975).
7 A. KILHAM, L., MARGOLIS, G.: Transmission of rat virus in milk of rats. J. infect. Dis. **129**, 737—740 (1974).
8 A. MENGELING, W. L.: Porcine parvovirus: Frequency of naturally occurring transplacental infection and viral contamination of fetal porcine kidney cell cultures. Amer. J. vet. Res. **36**, 41—44 (1975).
9 A. MENGELING, W. L., CUTLIP, R. C., WILSON, R. A., PARKS, J. B., MARSHALL, R. F.: Fetal mummification associated with porcine parvovirus infection. J. Amer. vet. med. Ass. **166**, 993—995 (1975).

10 A. PARRIS, D. S., BATES, R. C.: Replication of bovine parvovirus in S-phase cells. Amer. Soc. Microbiol. Abstr. p. 213 (1974).

11 A. PARRIS, D. S., BATES, R. C.: Effect of bovine parvovirus on macromolecular synthesis in synchronized cells. Amer. Soc. Microbiol. Abstr. p. 245 (1975).

12 A. SINGER, I. I., TOOLAN, HELEN W.: Ultrastructural studies of H-1 parvovirus replication. I. Cytopathology produced in human NB epithelial cells and hamster embryo fibroblasts. Virology **65**, 40—54 (1975).

13 A. TATTERSALL, P. J., WARD, D. C., SHATKIN, A. J.: Sequence overlap between the structural polypeptides of the Minute Virus of Mice. Abstr. Third Int. Congr. Virology, Madrid, p. 183 (1975).

VIROLOGY MONOGRAPHS

VIROLOGY
MONOGRAPHS